WIDENING HORIZONS
OF
CHILD HEALTH

Widening Horizons of Child Health

A study of the medical health needs of children in England and Wales

by

Alfred White Franklin
M.A., M.B., B.Ch., F.R.C.P., F.C.S.T. (Hon.)

With the help of working party of the British Paediatric Association and the Royal College of General Practitioners

Published with the support of
The Joseph Rowntree Memorial Trust

MTP

Published by MTP Press Limited
St. Leonard's House
Lancaster, England.

The publishers wish to acknowledge the kind support of The Joseph Rowntree Memorial Trust, York, in the publication of this book.

ISBN 0 85200165 7

Printed in Great Britain by R. & R. Clark Ltd., Edinburgh

Contents

Members of the working party

The Royal College of General Practitioners

Dr Stuart Carne, M.B., F.R.C.G.P., D.C.H., Hon. Treasurer to the R.C.G.P., Senior Tutor in General Practice to the R.P.M.S., Hammersmith Hospital, London

Dr John Wright, M.B., B.Ch., F.R.C.S., F.R.C.G.P., D.C.H., Senior Lecturer, Department of Community Medicine and General Practice, University of Leeds

The British Paediatric Association

Dr Alfred White Franklin, M.B., B.Ch., F.R.C.P., Consulting Paediatrician to Saint Bartholomew's Hospital, London E.C.1

Dr Walter Henderson, M.D., F.R.C.P., D.C.H., Consulting Paediatrician to the County Hospital, York

Dr J. N. Montgomery, M.D., F.R.C.P., D.C.H., Paediatric Consultant to the General Hospital, Plymouth

The Society of Medical Officers of Health

Dr Dorothy Egan, F.F.C.M., M.R.C.S., L.R.C.P., D.P.H., Hon. Consultant Paediatrician, Guy's Hospital, London S.E.

The Working Party has had the benefit of advice and encouragement from a number of members of the staff of the Department of Health and Social Security and from Dr Joyce Wetherall of the Office of Population Censuses and Surveys. Their kindness does not involve them or their departments in any responsibility for the views expressed in the book.

Foreword

The pattern of child health in Britain is changing, and paediatrics—the medicine of the dependent developing child—is changing too. What are the needs of children and expectation of parents today? And what kind of professional services are necessary to meet them effectively and with mutual satisfaction?

This book began in the enquiries and discussions of a working party set up in 1968 by the Royal College of General Practitioners and the British Paediatric Association.

The members came early to the conclusion that if the information available from national data and from local studies was more fully used needs could be more accurately measured and the relevant services more clearly seen.

As they followed this road, significant changes were taking place elsewhere: family medicine began to be seriously included in undergraduate education; the Royal Colleges and Associations accepted their responsibilities for vocational training; a radical reorganization of the National Health Service began; and Government set up a special committee to review the health services for children. In this new context the members decided to limit themselves to the changing pattern of health and disease in children: to illustrate how the paediatrics of illness was widening to include the paediatrics of development, of behaviour, of education, of family interaction and of social response.

Only when this was recognized they felt could a rational change in services and the training of those working in them take place. Those taking part felt their thinking and conclusions should be shared, their convener became their amanuensis and this book is the outcome. It is the view of a group of doctors caring for children shaped and focused by a paediatrician of great experience and wide sympathy. It is incomplete, and neither crosses the frontiers of its commitment nor evades the constraint of rapidly increasing knowledge and administrative change. Yet within and beyond the widening horizons can be glimpsed the implications for services and for the better training of practitioner and paediatrician in the care of children.

It is clear to us that such training cannot be confined within the walls of a university hospital but must spread into family practice, district hospitals and community services. The process has started in some medical schools, and general practitioners and paediatricians find they are natural allies in pressing for its extension.

This book is addressed primarily to doctors involved in the care of children, but it has much to say to other professional colleagues, nurses, health visitors, therapists and social workers who share the common task. Although neither an official publication of the College, nor of the Association, we, the Presidents of these bodies, are most grateful to the working party for their endeavours. We see their publication as another expression of our recognition of the need for shared responsibility in improving the health of children. We wish their publication well.

S. D. M. COURT
President
British Paediatric Association

P. S. BYRNE
President
Royal College of General Practitioners

January 1976

Acknowledgements

The origins in 1968 of the project which led to this study are briefly described in the first chapter. Through the operation of time and seniority of membership I was then President of the British Paediatric Association and so *ex officio* a member of the joint working party appointed by the Association and the Royal College of General Practitioners. The working party spent two years deciding what contribution it could usefully make and through the operation of time once more, because I left the National Health Service in 1970, I was able to accept the directorship of the Project.

My first acknowledgement must be to the constituent bodies, and then to the members of the working party for their thoughtful comment and criticism, for their help in gathering the basic material and for producing the skeleton which, once the stage of study was over, I was as Director invited to clothe.

In writing the Report I have had the opportunity to learn a great deal from the relevant literature, which is vast and which includes much about incidence and prevalence that I should have known in earlier years. I have also been lucky enough to have many lessons from and illuminating exchanges of views with experts too numerous to mention individually. Any of them who read this book will, I hope, accept my very real gratitude for their instruction and help. The views expressed owe much to others but the responsibility for them remains my own.

To have lived with the project for the five years that passed before the draft report was ready for circulation has been a great burden to my family whose forbearance has earned my wonder and my gratitude, now publicly recorded. The length of time has also meant that the 1969 figures current in the beginning had to be updated first to 1970 and then to 1971. When these figures became available the working party called a halt. In fact there is a curious consistency in patterns of prevalence and I hope that no critic will dismiss the contents as 'out-of-date' without doing his homework and comparing the latest figures published by 1975 when the draft was finished.*

The report could not have been prepared without the able help of

*RGSR for 1972 was published in 1974, and for 1973 in 1975. HIPE latest is for 1972 published in 1974.

Mrs Larrington at the Royal College of General Practitioners. My thanks are due to her as well as to Mrs Frances Robinson who laboriously typed the manuscript and to my own secretary Mrs Lora Russel.

Above all I am grateful to the Joseph Rowntree Memorial Trust whose confidence in the value of the study, inspired at first by Dr Walter Henderson, has been maintained to the point of their now undertaking its publication.

ALFRED WHITE FRANKLIN

Abbreviations

A.S.M.E.	Association for the Study of Medical Education.
B.P.A.	British Paediatric Association.
D.E.S.	Department of Education and Science.
D.H.S.S.	Department of Health and Social Security.
I.C.D.	International Classification of Diseases.
L.A.A.M.O.	Local Authority Assistant Medical Officer.
R.C.G.P.	Royal College of General Practitioners.
S.D.	Standard deviations.

CHAPTER 1

Introduction

To quantify the medical health needs of children would be impossible were academic accuracy required. Approximate estimates, recognized as such, have the practical value of showing what bulks largest in service requirements, whether preventive measures could reduce those requirments, where standards of service need most to be improved, especially for less serious but commonly occurring problems, and what conditions require either an inordinate amount of time or a high degree of expertise. But while the aim of this survey was to define service demands so that they might be in the end satisfied, its immediate purpose is to influence the content of the training programme for the general practitioner, the community orientated medical officer and the consulting, and indeed any other variety of, paediatrician.

Many other professionals are concerned with the promotion and the maintenance of the health of children, the health visitor, the social worker, the school nurse, the educational welfare officer, and the school teacher among them. And in the long run children depend for their health on those hard-working amateurs, parents. Although much of what is written in this book should be helpful to all of them and some of it especially to those concerned with children who have particular health needs, the target is the doctor with direct clinical responsibility towards children and their families and those who plan his education and training.

THE ORIGINS OF THE PROJECT

In October 1968 a symposium on Paediatric Education was organized by the BPA under the auspices of ASME. One result was the formation, at the suggestion of Lord Hunt of Fawley, of a working party of the BPA and the RCGP to examine what part the general practitioner should play in fulfilling the medical health needs of children.

During the early meetings, Dr John Wright persuaded the working party that the first step should be to make a quantitative estimate of these needs. He believed that much of the information was available and that the presentation of a coherent picture of the diseases, the disorders and the handicaps of children only awaited a patient search through existing reports. To gather all the information between the two covers of a book would help those planning paediatric education as well as those providing the necessary service.

After long discussion the working party with the agreement of the two constituent bodies decided to limit its survey to defining and as far as possible quantifying the medical health needs of children. This done the working party could consider how the information should influence the professional training of doctors. Meanwhile the Royal College of General Practitioners has formed its own conclusions about the general practitioner's role in the care of children and the paediatric content of vocational training, matters referred to in Chapter 11.

Dr Walter Henderson was fortunate in securing financial help from the Joseph Rowntree Memorial Trust, and in July 1970 the Director of the Project on Medical Health Needs of Children was appointed.

BACKGROUND TO THE STUDY

To survey and to do no more than form a quantitative estimate of disease, disorder and handicap would make dull and indigestible reading. It would also produce a misleading picture of what needs to be done. The quality of the need has therefore been examined and this reveals how great is the variety of necessary skills.

The Thousand Families Study in Newcastle upon Tyne, as it progressed, adopted a novel classification of diseases which included immunizing diseases, endemic family infections, diseases of social environment, disorders of development, and because of their great frequency, the respiratory diseases.

The classification, with its socio-economic and epidemiological insights, shed light on important factors in aetiology and pointed the way to possible preventive measures. It also defined to a great extent the function to be performed by the doctor in primary care. Twenty-five years have passed since the birth of the children enlisted for that study, a period that has seen undreamed of advances both in diagnostic and in therapeutic techniques. A complete National Health Service has been born and has come of age, and its cost in monetary and human resources has increased to the point where their unplanned consumption is unlikely to be possible for much longer.

As a background to the present survey a fresh classification of the medical health needs of children has been delineated. If the function of paediatrics is to ensure the fullest possible development of the child to the limit of his potential and to prevent what is preventable, the paediatrics of sickness recedes from its historic dominance, making room for the paediatrics of development, the paediatrics of education, the paediatrics of life and habit, psycho-paediatrics and the paediatrics of public health. To these should be added preventive paediatrics.

An appreciation of these titles, which in general reflect different facets of the health needs of children with medical problems, should not prevent the doctor from looking upon his child patient as a whole person. He has, too, to bear in mind that the child is part of a family and that the family remains the unit of society. The desired 'fullest development of the child to the limits of his potential' is only possible within the context of adequate family life.

SEVEN PAEDIATRIC FACETS OF CHILD HEALTH NEED

Children's needs for medical care can be examined from seven points of view. The proposed list is designed to promote the relevant training of personnel and the division of labour among them. Because the needs of the child are inter-related, the edges of the facets are not clean cut. Ideally one doctor would be sufficiently skilful to cover all these needs and any departure from management by one doctor has obvious disadvantages. Some doctors, unmindful of the importance of aptitude and training in satisfying the various needs, do feel compelled to tackle everything, but with the complexity of present health needs and of the means of supplying them, the idea that one doctor can manage everything is no longer tenable.

If it be true that under modern conditions the paediatrics of sickness recedes from its historic dominance, it is because the doctor increasingly recognizes the importance to health of these other aspects and of his need to appreciate them even if he cannot provide the therapeutic service himself. The seven points of view or facets are described as forms of paediatrics in the following way.

1 *The paediatrics of sickness* – care of the sick child

This includes the primary care of acute disease and accident, the treatment of chronic and recurrent disease and of congenital defect with particular attention to resulting physical disability, and with full understanding of the emotional disturbance and the delay in development that may result.

2 *The paediatrics of development* – care of the handicapped child

This aims at the earliest possible identification of handicap, especially of neuro-developmental handicap, and can only be based on familiarity with normal development. Suspicion that arises during perinatal care or surveillance of infants and young children should lead to attempts at comprehensive assessment. Understanding of the total health problem opens the way for treatment of the defect and for parent counselling and support. Some of the sequelae can be prevented and the harmful effects of what cannot be prevented can be minimized. In these ways the child can be helped to achieve maximum development of potential.

Appropriate community provision for education, training and recreation lead up to vocational guidance in relation to the handicap.

3 *The paediatrics of education* – the care of the child at school

School attendance and progress are affected by inadequacy of the family as well as by ill health or physical handicap of the pupil. School failure may result from specific learning disabilities such as defects of language, communication and perception, and motor defects, fine as well as gross. Defects of character and deficiencies of home environment also embarrass education.

4 *The paediatrics of life and habit* – the care of the child at home

The basic problem here may be environmental, familial or within the child himself. For example environmental hazards (dwellings, apparatus, damp, dangerous play space) predispose to accident, an important cause of morbidity and mortality. Family problems include adoption, illegitimacy, unmarried pregnancy, single parenthood, deprivation, including financial, nutritional and emotional deprivation, and child abuse. Reactions by the individual, i.e. 'bad habits', include overeating, drug, alcohol and smoking dependence, and delinquency.

5 *Psycho-paediatrics* – the mental health of the family

This title means something different from psychiatry applied to children, which must remain the responsibility of the psychiatrist. The three main components are first mental subnormality, secondly emotional maladjustment both primary and secondary and the counselling of parents and families in relation to mourning, rejection, the stress of handicap, guilt, over and under anxiety, and thirdly the effects of such family stress upon healthy sibling.

6 *The paediatrics of public health* – a safer society for the child

The five previous aspects of need concern the child and the family with a paediatric problem, of sickness or handicap. The environment can be improved to the benefit of all by the control of epidemics both in the community and in institutions, and by immunization programmes. Measures for the prevention of accident can also be taken by the community. Traditional public hygiene deals with health education and with the regulation of water supply, drainage, waste disposal and burial; and more recently the prevention of dental caries can be attempted by the fluoridation of water. Included also is knowledge of society's contribution to child health and to the understanding and the management of family problems through non-medical personnel such as social workers and health visitors.

7 *Preventive paediatrics*

The important theme of prevention should inform the whole of paediatrics. The prevention of the acute specific fevers or of dental caries, are included in the paediatrics of public health. Secondary prevention, for example the early identification of hearing defects so as to avoid delayed or absent development of speech, comes into the province of the paediatrics of development.

The urgency of prevention of disease and disorder varies directly with the seriousness of the condition and of its possible consequences. But it also depends on the efficacy and the availability of therapeutic measures. Where these are judged satisfactory, the impulse to search out preventive measures weakens. To take a simple example, congenital hypertrophic pyloric stenosis is now well recognized, seldom neglected, almost always successfully treated. Anyone who wanted to undertake a research into the prevention of this relatively common and benign abnormality would risk a reputation for eccentricity. By contrast, a few conditions, and those not of grave import such as obesity, urinary infections and anaemia in middle childhood appear in the quantitative estimates to occupy a great deal of medical and health service time. The argument could be sustained that this expenditure itself merits serious study with a view to more effective prevention.

Prevention—new style. Recent techniques have given a new meaning to prevention, enlarging its scope in several directions, all of which bring medical practitioners face to face with problems on the one hand of ethics and on the other of expenditure. In both the doctor is compelled to make decisions and to take actions which deeply commit his individual patients and their families as well as society as a whole. Organ transplants, amniocentesis, a new approach to abortion, the total care of babies with spina bifida cystica, the detection and destruction of abnormal products of conception, serve as examples.

It is sometimes claimed that doctors are 'dedicated as a profession to preserving life as long as possible and to dealing energetically with each threatening illness and each successive complication'.* By whose authority the doctors act is far from clear. That such dedication is not always in the best interests of the patient, the family or society is now a view openly discussed as what is called the 'quality of life' assumes more importance. The concept of always preventing the preventable is no longer accepted as axiomatic.

These value judgements have the look about them of professional arrogance as if doctors were the arbiters of fate, compelling their patients to survive 'as long as possible', knowing what are 'the best interests' of another human being and deciding the standard below which 'the quality of life' is too poor to be permitted. The compulsion to total treatment at whatever cost is balanced by the concept of euthanasia and easier access to termination of pregnancy. The aim of these two manoeuvres could be to protect man's genetic heritage, to save expense, to prevent suffering, or to satisfy the doctors professional pride or some emotional need of his which cannot be rationally expressed. It is certainly not to preserve life.

Nature has a method of correcting her own mistakes, if congenital defects which seriously impair and limit the development of an individual's fully adult potential may be regarded as mistakes. The mongol baby has a greater than normal liability to duodenal atresia and severe congenital heart disease. One in five stillbirths (RGSR for 1971) and 1401 or 18 per cent of the 7750 children who died in the first week of life, had a severe congenital anomaly. The contribution to miscarriage and spontaneous abortion made by genetic faults capable of causing severe anatomical defects can only be guessed.

Once the baby has been delivered with a beating heart, the neonatologist's dedication to preserving its life by all available means can be readily understood. He has a vested professional interest in success as well as in ensuring that threatened complications are foreseen and avoided. Technological advances and greater knowledge of the special physiology and pathology of the newborn baby, and especially of the premature baby, have undoubtedly increased the chances of undamaged survival in obstetric departments of excellence. How far the community will be able to raise general care to such standards remains to be seen.

*This quotation was copied verbatim from a paper given at a conference on organ transplantation, but unfortunately its provenance was not noted at the time. I cannot now find it, but I preserve it here because it expresses so aptly one point of view.

Meanwhile the importance is increasingly recognized of taking into account the circumstances under which the baby for salvage will live, socio-economic as well as emotional, in the life of the family into whose care he will go.

While the need to solve these vital problems becomes more urgent, much remains to be done to apply to the care of children the lessons already learned. The new enterprises, which aim to make the wellbeing of future generations a true and sincere priority, can never be completely successful. Their demand for trained personnel and their heavy cost impose limitations, which will call for sacrifices and for the acceptance of some scale of priorities. Nevertheless, the effort is surely worth making even though one area of sacrifice will certainly be the liberty of the practitioner always and only to recommend what suits his nature, his philosophy and his, necessarily limited, experience. Such a sacrifice is better made freely and by the light of reason than by even the most elegantly camouflaged direction.

Doctoring—new style

Team work. The idea behind this suggested classification is to light up the importance of team work, necessitated by the different facets of child health needs and the different medical approaches appropriate for their fulfilment. For example, a newborn baby, stressed at delivery and suffering from a neurological deficit, will first need the paediatrics of sickness and certainly the family will need psycho-paediatrics. The paediatrics of development and of education will later be brought into play. The child who needs all these aids for his own development and for his parents' emotional adjustment, may not receive them all from one kind of 'paediatrician'. The scheme of things must take account of the fact that one paediatrician may lack vocation or aptitude for some types of practice and many of the child's needs may require the services of other members of health care teams.

Neither the paediatrician nor the general practitioner can produce every solution single handed. The apparatus of child health care, as of family care of which child health care forms an integral part, includes midwives, health visitors, both community and hospital orientated social workers, school nurses and educational welfare officers. The part played by voluntary charitable societies must not be overlooked. The acceptance as important aetiological factors in disorders of child health of unsuitable housing, unemployment, the inadequacy, the delinquency or the psychopathy of parents, and of marital problems, enlarges the team still more. Resources of personnel and of money are unlikely ever to be sufficient, because in matters of health supply always creates demand. Demand never of itself creates supply and the shortfall will mirror exactly how much priority is honestly given in our society to provision for child health needs. It is of the greatest importance, therefore, to make the best use of what is available.

Team work, once its need is accepted, demands first that each member of the team understands and values the expertise of the others. Communication between members of the team must be free and frank. Above all the team members should not attempt to do each other's work. Exclusiveness and professional arrogance must be foresworn.

Hospital or community based? In the construction of this report a relatively small proportion of space is occupied by the needs of children for hospital in-patient care. This is not because such work is lightly regarded, but rather because the widening of the health horizon has changed the nature of the needs. The paediatrician continues to find the care of sick children in hospital a major avocation. So do the therapeutic experts, medical and surgical, who concentrate their attention on systems and organs. Improved treatments enable the general practitioner now to undertake safely at home the primary care of many of the children suffering from the acute infections. The home itself has attained qualities which make it a safer environment than at any previous time in recent history for the treatment of acute illness, and social policy allows many adaptations for the disabled and the chronic sick.

An even smaller proportion of space is given to the work done in the out-patient departments. This results from the absence of any central records of what happens there. Some form of classification of this invaluable work is desirable, not least because the development of 'clinic' diagnosis would benefit the Health Service and the children by decreasing the number of hospital admissions, and by leading the way to a more rational use of hospital doctors' time. What can and what cannot be accomplished in 'out-patients' needs to be surveyed with a view to more effective staffing and organization. Out-patient departments deserve as much thoughtful design and planning as wards. That the advisability is generally accepted of separating children from adults in out-patients as well as in the wards is taken for granted.

The reorganization of the National Health Service with its concept of Health Areas should make possible studies of this kind. Both for management and for undergraduate teaching of the medical student, the out-patient clinic must assume more of the value now given to the hospital bed and the community itself must attract much of the attention now paid to the hospital. The aim must be for the child to obtain its medical care, preventive, diagnostic and therapeutic, under appropriate circumstances and in the most suitable place. An element of choice must remain, but the element of chance which bears so much responsibility for unevenness and at times for inadequacy of care, should be reduced to the minimum. The training of the doctors of the future must also take place in the most appropriate environment.

CHAPTER 2

Sources

This survey concerns children from birth to the end of the fourteenth year in England and Wales unless otherwise stated. The Working Party decided not to try to quantify the medical health problems of adolescence to which attention is drawn occasionally. Only when some practical purpose is served are the sexes considered separately. Differences undoubtedly exist between different parts of the two countries and between urban and rural populations. The Working Party, having discussed these differences, decided against the attempt to illustrate them because of their complexity.

DIAGNOSED AND NAMED DISEASE

The main sources of general information are

The Registrar General's Statistical Review for England and Wales 1971 (RGSR)
Report on Hospital In-Patient Enquiry 1971 (HIPE)
Morbidity Statistics from General Practice, second national study 1970–71 (GPR)

Important studies based on special populations which have been consulted and which are described below include

Observations by J. W. B. Douglas and co-workers on a 1948 Cohort
The Thousand Families Study in Newcastle upon Tyne, based on a 1947 Cohort
The National Children's Bureau Studies in Child Development based on a 1958 Cohort (NCB)
The Isle of Wight Studies on 1964 and 1965 Cohorts (IOW).

Reference is made in the appropriate place to many reports on special diseases and disorders and to the Department of Education and Science's Statistics of Education (1970).

The International Classification of Disease is referred to in the text as ICD.

THE SOURCES OF INFORMATION

The Registrar-General's Statistical Review

The modern interest in medical and vital statistics began in England in the late seventeenth century with the work of Sir William Petty and John Graunt (Greenwood 1948). More than a century and a half before the establishment of the General Register Office, Petty proposed a register of births, marriages, burials, houses, the ages, sexes and occupation of the people so that 'his Majesty may have a yearly account of the encrease and decrease of his Subjects' (Lansdowne 1927). Petty's interests in the state of the nation extended widely into trade, customs and excise, scholarship, the law, prisoners and executions. He saw a need to know the numbers of live and still births and of abortions, of admissions to and discharges from 'hospitals, Bedlam, orphans' each month and to know when an epidemic of plague was appearing. In London, 'when 100 per week dy, the Plague is begun'. The inhabitants of London, where in 'pestilential yeares' one sixth of the people 'dy', should then be evacuated at seven days' notice to a circle of 70 miles diameter from the centre. This should cut deaths by one half.

The purpose of Petty's quantification was essentially practical and some of it was directly medical. The statistical information had therefore to be not only as accurate as possible but also as readily available as possible. He would not have been satisfied with the appearance of compilations one or two years after the events which are computed. His interest centred in London with its 134 parishes, 800 000 people, 120 000 families and 108 000 houses. The census of 1831 showed that the population of England and Wales had risen from 8 872 980 in 1801 to 13 894 574 so that already analyses were bound to take more and more time. It was no longer 'his Majesty' who needed the information. An Act for Registering Births, Deaths and Marriages in England, of the 6th and 7th of William IV, 'required the Registrar-General to send once in every year to one of the principal Secretaries of State a General Abstract of the Number of Births, Deaths, and Marriages during the foregoing year' to be laid before Parliament. So began the annual reports with volume one for the year ending 30 June 1838, being the first year of Registration under the Act and published for Her Majesty's Stationery Office in 1839.

In the introduction the Registrar-General noted differences in vital statistics between town and country and between different areas of England. He also observed that 'if a watch or a machine is destroyed by dashing it upon the ground or throwing it into the fire, its motion may also be arrested by internal causes having their source in its own mechanism'. Commenting that the 'diseases enumerated in the first London Bills of Mortality did not exceed 65' and referring to the greater number described in later nosologies, he concludes that 'The primary divisions of a *Statistical Nosology* should evidently be founded upon the mode in which diseases affect the population'. Epidemic, endemic and contagious diseases, of which 27 are listed, were of major importance accounting for more than one fifth of all deaths analyzed. Smallpox contributed about 5 per cent of these deaths. The sporadic diseases were classified by Systems such as 'nervous system and senses', organs of respiration, of circulation, eleven in all and in a general pattern that has altered but little since. Each class contains a number of sub-headings. The last class, 'of uncertain seat', includes among its sub-headings many of paediatric concern, rickets, scurvy, atrophy, malformations, cyanosis or blue disease, imperforate anus and 'spina bifida etc.'. There were 335 956 registered deaths during the year and 399 712 births and miscarriages. In the half-year analyzed for cause of death 1265 women had died in child-bed, mostly from puerperal fever.

The Registrar-General's Statistical Review of England and Wales replaced this Abstract following the Census Act 1920 which required him 'to collect and publish any available statistical information with respect to the number and condition of the population in the interval between one census and another'. In presenting the review for the year 1921 in the first volume of the new series (1923) the Registrar-General expressed the desire to improve the value and instructiveness of the medical and civil statistics by additions and 'by eliminating matter which appeared to have outlived its real utility'. At that time the total population was 37 885 242 with 457 678 deaths including 112 906 under 15 years old compared with, fifty years later, 48 894 500, with 567 262 total deaths and 18 516 deaths in childhood. The births in 1921 numbered 848 814, 38 618 of them illegitimate, compared with 783 155 total births in 1971 of which 65 678 were illegitimate, almost twice the proportion. Deaths in 1921 numbered 70 250 (83 per 1000 births) in the first year, 29 932 under 4 weeks of which 9150 occurred on the first day. This compares with 13 720 deaths in the first year (74 per cent), 9112 under 4 weeks (49 per cent) including 4680 on the first day (25 per cent). The number of children of school age (5 to 14) has changed little, 7 407 273 in 1921 compared with 7 756 600 in 1971.

What has changed almost out of recognition has been the nosology. The two directions of change are the numbers of possible diagnoses and concepts of the nature of disease. 'The number of individual diseases and syndromes', wrote Reichertz (1973), 'has increased from 5000 to about 30 000 since the turn of the century, and will probably increase still further.' Much depends on the angle from which the diseased patient is viewed. In bacterially produced disease what should be the determinant in classification? Should it be the specific organism, the site at which clinical evidences are recognized, or, when they are identified, immunological deficiences or socio-economic hazards? As far as children are concerned, there were in 1971 four classes of major causes of death—perinatal conditions (33 per cent), congenital anomalies (19.5 per cent), diseases of the respiratory system (16.5 per cent) and accidents, poisonings and violence (11.7 per cent). The remaining thirteen classes contain between them less than one fifth (19 per cent).

The death rate of children below the age of one year in 1971 was 18 per thousand live births, following a steady downward course. A decline to zero would not appear to be realistic. At what point can it be accepted that the lowest reasonable figure has been reached? To consider the fate of the conceptus rather than that of the newborn baby opens up possibilities of following nature's method of aborting imperfections. A combination of ideal obstetrics and perfect prediction of fetal abnormality would in theory produce a considerable increase in the perinatal survival rates of undamaged babies. Perinatal conditions and congenital anomalies together account for 52.5 per cent of childhood deaths and for much morbidity besides.

The reactions of the upper and lower respiratory tract to attack from without and to stress from within needs much more study before rational prophylaxis becomes possible. Successful prophylaxis would accomplish a great reduction in the work of doctors, something that is to be deduced from all the available morbidity studies. Fewer childhood deaths mean more old people with degenerative diseases. Nevertheless to reduce mortality in infancy and childhood as well as morbidity must be accepted as important to child health needs. Accident, which contributes to both, is always assumed to be preventable and here again more needs to be learnt about aetiological factors. Valuable information is given in the tables listing the incidents by the external cause, the nature of the injury and as non-transport accidents, road traffic accidents and accidents in the home.

The Registrar-General's Annual Statistical Review could provide more useful information about Child Health Needs by adopting the Juvenile Diagnostic List instead of ICD based on disease in adults. Even then there would be limitations. Few perinatal deaths result from a single factor. In reports prepared by obstetric hospitals and departments this has always been a source of difficulty, since for practical purposes the important pieces of information required are: which of all the adverse factors is the critical one and what was the time of its operation. Improvements as opposed to changes in both obstetric and paediatric techniques depend upon this kind of knowledge. The necessary flexibility is unlikely to fit any form of static tabulation. This is, *par excellence*, the place for on-going computer analysis. Neonatal deaths in the first week of life are tabulated for the calculation of perinatal death rates. Of immense value would be a detailed study of the first four weeks which included the results of social enquiry as well as all the other possible aetiological factors.

Report on Hospital In-Patient Enquiry

This enquiry was designed primarily to aid administration. The two methods are, first, to provide information in terms of diseases treated and (some of) the characteristics of patients who had those diseases, such as age and sex, and, second, to provide data relating to 'the amount, distribution and effect of illness in the community and various sections of it'. The resulting figures are estimates of total discharges from hospital or deaths in hospital, based on a report of every tenth case multiplied by a calculated factor. The International Classification of Disease is used, the case being assigned to the principal condition treated. This is considered preferable to the use of the presenting symptom or leading sign and more practicable or at least more consistent than the use of the underlying cause. Unfortunately most classes contain large entries of 'unspecified' conditions. The study of child health needs limits the use of the enquiry to those tables which are age-related and it must always be borne in mind that the figures do not represent patients but discharges and deaths. Neither the duration of stay nor the regional distribution tables have been utilized. A detailed consideration of the HIPE data is to be found in Chapter 10.

Morbidity Statistics from General Practice, second national study 1970–71

Two national studies of morbidity statistics from general practice in England and Wales have been undertaken by the General Practice Research Unit of the Royal College of General Practitioners, the first 1955–56 and the second, which has been used for this survey, in 1970–71.

The Registrar-General's Review is concerned with all registered deaths and the In-Patient Enquiry with a selected group of discharges from and deaths in hospital. The GP statistics fill an obvious gap in knowledge of the GP's work but are limited to a selection of practices and concern the morbidity not of the population but of those who decide to consult their general practitioner. Information is also collected about the extent to which family doctors use health facilities outside their practices.

The records were made in 53 practices, mostly with lists of 2000 to 4000 per principal serving a population of 292 247, and involved 118 doctors. Of particular importance for the medical care of children is the large proportion of single-handed practices in the study, 23 or 43 per cent, which is the national proportion. There were only nine partnerships of four or more, 17 per cent, slightly higher than the national figure (14.2 per cent). The fact that the greater part of the child population will be consulting a truly general practitioner gives an even greater importance to paediatrics in his vocational training, something well recognized by the College.

The child population in the study totalled 69 748, which is no more than about 1 in 167 of the total child population 0 to 14 years in 1971. The proportion of males to females matches, but the distribution in the two age groups, 0–4 and 5–14 years, differs a little. Under-fives, who need the most attention, form 33.5 per cent of the general child population but only 30.9 per cent of the practice children in the study. While the small numbers in the study do not provide a basis for extrapolation to the general population, they are big enough to give an important insight into the reasons for which children are taken to general practitioners and into the numbers referred by them for further medical service.

Valuable also is the comparison between the proportions within each ICD class in a general practice and in hospital work. For example Class XVI of the International Classification contains 17 headings (780–796) for symptoms and ill-defined conditions. In the General Practitioner survey these have enough sub-headings to multiply nearly four times to 67 and the class contributes 24.8 per cent of all childhood consultations. By contrast Class XVI in HIPE contributes 7.9 per cent (6154 out of 78 044) and among RGSR deaths only 1.7 per cent (320 out of 18 517).

These childhood consultations are for a mixture of symptoms and signs which have been labelled rather than diagnosed, for example cough consultations amount to 4168, 33.5 per cent, and acute vomiting and/or diarrhoea to 3602, 29.0 per cent, totalling 62.5 per cent of the whole class.

Data from this study are discussed in Chapter 11.

Studies by J. W. B. Douglas and co-workers

In 1946 the Population Investigation Committee began a survey of the economic and social facts of childbirth. During one week in March,

13 687 babies were enrolled in 424 maternity and child welfare areas in all parts of England and Wales and from all social classes. The Director, Dr J. W. B. Douglas, supported in the belief that the opportunity was too good to miss, has continued his observations on 12 930 legitimate single births, having excluded multiple and illegitimate pregnancies. These observations have been published as 'Children under Five' (JWBD and J. M. Blomfield 1958), 'The Home and the School' (JWBD 1964) and 'All our Future' (JWBD, J. M. Ross and H. R. Simpson 1968). The children in the long-term survey are all those born to wives of non-manual workers and farm labourers and one quarter of those born to wives of other types of manual workers and the self-employed with the exclusion of multiple and illegitimate births. The residual total comprises 5386 children. The orientation of these studies is educational combined with an attempt to correlate disturbed behaviour, educational disappointment and delinquency with the influence of the home and family. Not surprisingly pre-school care emerges as an important factor. In interpreting results two important facts must be remembered. In 1946, before the National Health Service, few newborn babies received specialized care from paediatricians and, secondly, since 1946 the prevention and treatment of neonatal infection have been revolutionized. Survival of a 1946 cohort of premature babies depended more on the competence of the baby than of its treatment.

The Thousand Families Studies in Newcastle upon Tyne

This enterprise, brain child of Sir James Spence, aimed to describe the pattern of disease during childhood. Begun in 1947 before the National Health Service and in the early days of antibiotic treatment, the investigation has changed with the resulting change in paediatric outlook. Much can be learned about the pattern of diseases in its family context despite these changes and the results show the urgent need for a reorientation of teaching in the subjects of paediatrics and child health.

'Growing up in Newcastle upon Tyne', the second volume (Miller *et al.* 1960) described the extent as well as the pattern of illness during early childhood in Newcastle upon Tyne. The main purposes of the enquiry at this time were to discuss the frequency and types of illness seen in a representative group of young children and to show that the occurrence and natural history of illness can be understood only if regarded as an aspect of the community in which it occurs. When illness develops in a growing child the patterns of outcome are influenced by the child's environment as well as by the particular agents of infection or of injury.

In the final volume, 'The School Years in Newcastle upon Tyne 1952–62' (Miller *et al.* 1974) attention is drawn to the altered underlying concept. The interest now centres on measured performance in relation to measured environment. The chief determinants of performance, biological growth, injury and disease, social adaptation and educational attainment, are 'so interrelated that separation even for classification and description, brings a sense of artificiality'. The authors claim that 'doctors must enlarge their concept of medicine to include the management and prevention of social and educational, as well as physical disease'. While no-one can dispute the doctor's claim to diagnostic skills and his need to recognize social and educational factors, the part which he is capable of playing directly in the management of social and educational 'disease' is open to question. Even in prevention his role may be perforce limited to the identification of the family at risk and the vulnerable child. Where the doctor's responsibility ends and to whom he then passes it are matters for serious study and for inclusion in any complete curriculum.

The present study of child health needs provides incontrovertible evidence of the changes necessary for the wider education of children's health teams and of all those doctors who work with children. Membership of the health team is not less important for the teachers charged with the responsibility of pre-school, infant and junior school education. As to the social worker, an essential step now is to gather and to apply all available knowledge, not only about the development of children and assessment of progress but also about the nature of the special problems of family life at the stage when the family itself is growing. It is difficult to believe that the best care can be planned and delivered without specialization.

The National Child Development Study (1958 *cohort*)

All the births in one week of March 1958 in England and Wales as well as in *Scotland* formed a cohort which was originally studied to enable observations to be made on the influences of pregnancy and perinatal factors on the health and development of a population of children. This cohort has fortunately been utilized for further investigation under the direction of the National Children's Bureau. The result has been a series of valuable publications which include data of incidence and prevalence. The sweep observations at seven years old have been published as 'From Birth to Seven' by R. Davie, N. Butler, H. Goldstein and co-workers. Data are identified as (NCB). Some 16 000 children are involved and child health is studied in its widest purview. Health and physical development, behaviour and adjustment, educational abilities and attainments are examined against a background of regional and social class differences. In interpreting comparisons with other data, the inclusion of Scotland must be remembered.

The Isle of Wight Surveys

These were carried out in 1964 on children aged 9 to 11 years and in 1965 on children aged 10 to 12 years in the Isle of Wight. The results were published under the title 'Education, Health and Behaviour' in 1970 by M. Rutter, J. Tizard and K. Whitmore referred to as (IOW). The aim of the studies was to consider service needs in relation to the prevalence of intellectual and educational retardation, psychiatric disorder and physical handicap. The children with handicaps, 'any disability which impedes the child in some way in his daily life', were compared with a randomly selected control group of children drawn from the general population. As with other surveys important associations are found between children's socio-familial background and the presence of handicap.

Special reports

A number of governmental, departmental and other reports on special subjects have been studied. Reference is made in the text under the name of either the chairman or the subject.

NON-PARTICIPANTS AND NON-DISEASE

Two other matters require attention if the potential workload of the doctor and a health service are to be measured. There is first the patient with a disease who fails to consult and second the patient with 'non-disease' who does. Butterfield in his survey in Bermondsey and Southwark (1968) showed that of the three quarters of the community studied who had complaints about health only one in four consulted a doctor at all. Of 2500 persons in a sample, 1000 were treating themselves, and of the remaining 1500 adults who took some action, 239 attended the general practitioner, 134 a local authority clinic, 71 a hospital, 54 a dentist, 45 non-medical help in the NHS and 6 an industrial medical organization. These figures do not represent children, for whom no similar study is available. Nevertheless many mothers who eventually attend hospital with their children have already taken advice from relatives, the local chemist and the health visitor before visiting the general practitioner's surgery. In any discussion of health needs of children in a total population, the problems of delivery of care are important. But it is of equal importance that the child with a health problem should identify himself. Much of child health need may still go unrecognized and so unmet. Surveillance services and immunization programmes never reach 100 per cent of the population and it would not be surprising to find the lowest rates of service usage among those families most in need. How to deliver health care to those who really need it is a challenge that must be met.

Turning to the patient with a 'non-disease', his positive recognition is often just as complex and expensive in time, personnel, apparatus and money, as is the establishment of a diagnosis. Clinical skill in the best hands must be better than it has ever been since the pathology of the living has both enlarged and enhanced the pathology of the post-mortem room. Nevertheless clinical confidence is weakened by the knowledge that diagnosis on clinical grounds alone takes second place to laboratory diagnosis, and even radiological diagnosis is giving way progressively to the direct inspection by fibreoptic endoscopy of more and more parts of the human body. One result of these refinements has been to make it increasingly difficult to exclude a disease diagnosis. The value of negative tests in stabilizing a clinical situation and restoring confidence is undeniably great. Yet the high proportion and great number of normal and negative test results bear witness to the extent of 'non-disease'.

While every patient who consults a doctor does so in the belief—usually a fear but sometimes a hope—that he has a medical problem, the larger proportion neither need nor benefit from a technological investigation in the laboratory or the x-ray department. They are not suffering from the kind of organ or system disease which such examinations can confirm. The general practitioner stands guard over the gateway to these tests and to the specialist consultant who uses them and who may indeed risk losing his reputation by not using all of them that are available.

In order to save time, money and the patient's comfort the validation, already being undertaken, of diagnostic techniques and the surest and least complicated methods of diagnosing 'non-disease' are seen to be urgent matters for study. Computer programmes should be capable of showing the ideal sequence for investigations and at which point in the chase pursuit is so likely to be fruitless that it may be safely abandoned.

CHAPTER 3

The first five years

NEONATAL ASSESSMENT

The objectives of the initial examination of the newborn baby are firstly, reassurance of the mother that her new baby appears to be completely normal but, if it does not, the early identification of abnormality. Secondly comes the institution of treatment directed against the abnormality itself and against all those additional problems that may result from the abnormality and whose effects can be minimized or prevented. The Infant At Risk Register aimed at the earliest possible delivery of medical care to infants in certain groups with a prediction of a higher than normal incidence of 'hidden handicaps', especially in the neuromuscular system. Recent discussions have led to a move away from the 'at risk' register mainly because it fails to achieve these objectives efficiently, and a move towards an initial assessment coupled with biochemical screening tests and followed by periodic surveillance of all babies. This should include help for normal babies.

The Peel Committee (1970) has recommended a paediatric examination of all newborns 'by a paediatric consultant or by a doctor who should be trained and experienced in the detection of deviations from the normal which call for urgent attention or surveillance' (para 272). This means the examination of at least a dozen new babies every day, taking little account of weekends and holidays. If paediatric examinations were made also by medical assistants, senior registrars and registrars, the daily load of new cases would be half a dozen. The matter might be somewhat complicated by the geographical distribution of the babies. Consultant cover cannot be provided for every newborn baby. Such skilled examination must be limited to those babies showing any suspicious symptoms or signs. The major part of neonatal assessment of the apparently normal will be carried out at the first attendance at the Child Health Centre or at the General Practice Centre. In either case, training in and experience of neonatal behaviour and physical examination must form an important element in training of both paediatricians and general practitioners. The needs of those who will practise obstetrics are also important. For this reason the total exclusion of obstetric staff from the care of the baby after delivery may not be in the best interests of child health since, with no direct responsibility for the baby's care, the obstetrician is in danger of regarding it as merely an object to be extracted from the mother as swiftly and as conveniently as possible.

The paediatrician should include in his responsibilities periodic reviews of the techniques of neonatal care. Technical advances in prevention and treatment have focused his interest on rhesus incompatibility, respiratory problems including the dangers of hypoxia, and improved care of small and early babies. His more general duty to ensure a healthy basis for the newborn baby's emotional development and to help the mother to make good adjustments to her baby may sometimes have been neglected. Ethological studies have shown the importance for both of early physical contact between mother and newborn baby. Only unequivocal medical reasons, of which there are few, should lead to interference with the natural course of events. There is no denying that failure to appreciate family reactions, as well as some traditional practice and much prejudice, still disturb this basis for the good emotional bonding which is as necessary for the mother as it is for the baby.

While total standardization of management techniques, including feeding and methods of prevention of infection, is not necessary, a recommendation from an authoritative source, generally acceptable to obstetricians, midwives and paediatricians, and not omitting mothers, is long overdue. These matters should also be reviewed by those in charge of general practitioner units in discussions with area consultants in obstetrics and paediatrics.

In the search for technical aids to prevent structural injury and to preserve life, the emotional needs and reactions of mother, father and baby run the risk of being overlooked. The students of both paediatrics and obstetrics should be instructed that the securing of the safe delivery of an unharmed baby and protection of the mother from injury and unnecessary suffering are the chief but not the sole objectives. The necessity for acceptance and integration of the new baby into the family must never be forgotten.

The concept of the fetus as a passive object to be expelled from the uterus to become a baby passively receiving impressions from the outside world is rapidly losing credibility. A hormonal contribution from the fetus plays some part in the initiation of labour. The organization of the central nervous system of the baby is now known to be more advanced than was believed in earlier times. The baby's behaviour and reactions, which influence emotional relationships, particularly with the mother, need to be observed, interpreted and heeded in programmes of management. The early interactions between mother and new baby may not last for life but they are undoubtedly of major importance for the future success of family life. Fortunately these aspects of neonatal life are now being scientifically studied.

SPECIAL CARE OF THE NEWBORN

A brief historical reminder of the development of the idea behind the provision of special care will focus attention on the present lack of any uniform philosophy and practice. Accurate quantification of need is, as a result, virtually impossible in terms of nursery accommodation and specialized staff. When babies were expected to be born at home, newborn babies were to be found in hospitals because of the obstetric problems of pregnant women. The babies remained with the mothers and the chief dangers were those of hospital infection. Small and premature babies were nursed in bathrooms, linen rooms, the offices of ward sisters, but only rarely did a hospital include special accommodation for babies.

The earliest changes were the provision of nurseries to which normal babies could be banished at night or by day if noisy and of the special nursery for the segregation of 'premature babies' so that nursing skill could be fostered in their feeding and management. Observations could be collected about their behaviour both in health and in disease, and relative freedom from infection ensured by isolation techniques. The sulpha drugs in the mid nineteen-thirties provided the second breakthrough in maternal mortality from puerperal infection some 85 years after Semmelweiss' first successful attack.

The control of neonatal infection, then the third commonest cause of neonatal mortality and morbidity, had to await the use of penicillin and the later antibiotics in the nineteen-forties. Meanwhile antenatal care improved, was better used and was more widely available. Obstetrical management also improved with midwives more highly trained and doctors better educated, all able to use the teachings of Eardley Holland and other pioneers in the mechanics of labour which had reduced the incidence of 'birth-deaths'. With the risks reduced of both gross trauma and infection, the remaining large problem of congenital defect could be studied more carefully. Possibilities of surgical treatment for congenital disorders of the alimentary tract and the cardiovascular system strengthened the need for more accurate and earlier diagnosis. Great advances were made during the late nineteen-forties coincidentally with better understanding and management of rhesus iso-immunization.

All these changes were occurring when the National Health Service made possible the general irruption into obstetrics of the paediatrician, who had previously functioned in only a few hospitals in England and

Wales. His need for a base in the hospital from which to operate combined with his need to study in detail the special physiology, pathology and management of the newborn baby produced an irresistible case for special nurseries.

Special care nurseries

One of the results has been some confusion about the purpose of special neonatal accommodation. Was it intended for the special treatment of sick newborn babies? Was it intended for the special care of premature or small-for-dates babies? As time passed and in accordance with the wish of obstetricians (Peel 1970), obstetrics became a hospital rather than a domiciliary process and experienced nursing staff failed to multiply at the same rate as the new hospitals. Was the special nursery to be used as the only safe observation ward for all or for special groups of neonates during their first few hours of life?

Meanwhile an authoritarian approach to childbirth which had insisted that babies should not be born at home led to attempts, once the place of birth had been determined, to organize the time of birth. There was too an implicit decision that no newborn baby should be allowed to die, at whatever expense in equipment, personnel, drugs and emotion. The obstetric nursery has in these ways come to serve many purposes in every hospital. In some all babies are admitted for the first few hours, in some only babies of 2500 g and less, and in others, only those in this weight range who present abnormal signs or symptoms and all those weighing 1500 g and less. Some hospitals, run on scientific and research orientated lines, well staffed, elaborately equipped and served by laboratory techniques of great sophistication, justly claim an increased survival of potentially normal babies. A heartless sceptic could ask whether these elaborate undertakings are justified, whether they make any notable impact on national statistics of mortality or later morbidity, and whether their methods are applicable to England and Wales as a whole. This is another example of the general ethical problem posed by highly skilful technology. When the first question, 'can something be done?', has been answered in the affirmative, the second question is 'should it be done?'

Meanwhile certain approximations can be reached. In 1971 6.0 per cent of all live born babies weighed 2500 g or less. Without separating the gestationally immature from the small-for-dates babies, the neonatal mortality rates for the babies of birthweight 2000 g and less were 300.5 per 1000 compared with 108.1 per 1000 of all infants of birth weight 2500 g and less and 12.3 per 1000 for all infants. Of babies of birthweight 2000 g and less, 67.5 per cent died in the first 24 hours (see Table 3.1).

It is estimated that 47 202 live newborn babies of 2500 g and less were born during 1971. Of the 5081 weighing 1500 g and less who would certainly have been admitted to special nursery 2021 had died within 24 hours of birth and only 2234 survived the first month. A population of 250 000 is expected to need one such special nursery of at least 24 cots. This means about 200 for England and Wales on a population basis, not allowing for geography (see Table 3.2).

The BPA recommendation is that the special care nursery should form part of the hospital children's department and should provide a training ground for neonatal medicine. The minimum medical staff should be the two consultant paediatricians, one member of the paediatric resident staff whose primary duty should be the special care nursery, three resident paediatric staff engaged solely in neonatal work, plus an additional sick children's resident for extra cover.

Apart from actual patient care, perinatal mortality and morbidity should be regularly reviewed and research work should be carried out.

If the estimate of 200 special care nurseries for England and Wales be correct, the minimum medical staffing alone would require 400 consultant paediatricians, 200 paediatric residents of registrar status, 600 resident paediatric staff working virtually full time. There would be also a high nursing staff to patient ratio during the whole 24 hours and the constant availability of pathology technicians. The general practitioner should be aware of the kind of work which can be carried on in such units. It is difficult to see what direct part he could be expected to play.

SCREENING FOR ENZYME AND METABOLIC DISORDERS

The idea that life-long disability results from anatomical defects of genetic origin is well established in medical, educational and administrative thinking. Recent technological advances in protein and enzyme chemistry and electron microscopy of lysosomes have provided explanations for many hitherto mysterious diseases, especially the 'storage diseases'. Some of the secondary effects of these metabolic faults are already preventable by dietary treatment, and with greater knowledge others may follow.

Because harmful variants provide chemical explanations for some forms of mental defect, detection must be early enough to precede the appearance of clinical manifestations and must take the form of screening examinations. The problems inherent in any screening system such as

Table 3.1. Notifications of low birth weight live and stillbirths by birth weight and mortality, 1971, England
(Annual Report of CMO, DHSS, for 1971, Table IX.4)

Birth weight group	*'Premature' live births*	*Deaths within 24 hours of birth*	*Deaths within 28 days of birth*	*Deaths within 28 days per 1000 live 'premature' births*	*'Premature' still births*	*'Premature' stillbirths per 1000 live and still 'premature' births*
–1000 g (–2 lb 3 oz)	1 803	1 062	1 442	799.7	1 156	390.7
–1500 g (–3 lb 4 oz)	3 278	959	1 432	436.8	1 515	316.1
–2000 g (–4 lb 6 oz)	8 375	707	1 170	139.7	1 404	143.6
–2250 g (–4 lb 15 oz)	10 452	267	503	48.1	642	57.9
–2500 g (–5 lb 8 oz)	23 294	262	550	23.6	692	28.9
All babies of 2500 g (–5 lb 8 oz) or less	47 202	3 257	5 097	108.1	5 409	102.8

Table 3.2. Number of babies requiring special care in 1969 in England and Wales

(estimated by the expert group on special care for babies, 1972)

(a)	Difficult deliveries		84 478
(b)	Live births 2500 g or less		53 419
(c)	Sick babies over 2500 g		
	ICD 760–3, 769–773 'sick'	31 197	
	ICD 754 Congenital heart	3000	
	ICD 764–8 Perinatal infections	4000	
			38 197
(d)	Later fetal deaths		7895

(HMSO Reports on Public Health and Medical Subjects No. 127)

false negatives and false positives have to be accepted as part of the human cost. The desirability and the scope of large-scale screening programmes have to be assessed against the expenditure of time, money and personnel, and the invasion of the liberty of the subject. Absolute quantification of many of the defects is not yet possible. Sir Archibald Garrod's expectation has been amply confirmed that there are many inborn variants in human metabolic processes and that alternative metabolic pathways do not necessarily result in disease. The distinction between variants which are actually or only potentially harmful and those that are harmless is by no means clear. Results to be valid involve the screening of geographical populations, or of special 'high risk' populations. For example conditions liable to be found among immigrants include glucose–6–phosphate dehydrogenase deficiency, haemoglobinopathy S and thalassaemia trait.

The criteria for population screening include the availability of at least three things: a simple and reliable screening method, specific tests for absolute confirmation, and treatment of proven value in preventing or limiting damage to tissues.

Dietary control may protect a vulnerable baby from the increasingly serious results of stress on an incomplete or abnormal metabolic pathway. The fetus exposed to a harmful intra-uterine environment in Rhesus incompatibility may be protected by the infusion into its peritoneum of compatible blood.

When treatment is unavailable and mental defect is certain or when a serious chromosomal abnormality is present, the logical preventive treatment consists of identification of the fetus at risk with the prospect of the termination of fetal life, a novel concept of prophylaxis from the viewpoint of the fetus doomed to destruction. Advantages accrue to the family, who are spared an abnormal child, and to the Health Service, which is saved the expense of treatment. Limiting the number of individuals carrying the abnormal genes is presumably an advantage for the population. What has yet to be determined is whether there are balancing disadvantages other than the occasional destruction, through some error of interpretation, of a potentially normal child. This outcome, the destruction of a fetus not known to be abnormal, is already accepted as justifiable if it is believed that the mother would benefit socially or in health and happiness. What is not yet certain is whether these ends are always secured by these means. Does a conscious decision to terminate a pregnancy at the end of the first trimester necessarily have long-term advantages over allowing the mother to complete her pregnancy and then destroying the baby if it were found to be abnormal? If we truly wish to exclude from our population as many people as we can with inherited and congenital defects, this question, as distasteful as it is unwelcome, may need to be faced and answered.

Some circumscribed populations must be intensively studied without delay so that accurate quantification does become possible. Racial origins must be recorded. Careful collation of long-term observations should reveal the natural history and the results of treatment, some of which may be damaging. The effect of the conscious choice of termination of pregnancy on total family health, both physical and emotional, must also be studied. Cold termination of pregnancy presents a different emotional problem from that of miscarriage or spontaneous abortion. Biological planning should not rest on prejudices and preconceived ideas.

New and improved techniques for the study of enzymes in blood plasma and in red and white cells, skin, mucosa, fibroblasts and amniotic cells and fluid, have made possible not only screening of the newborn, but for certain disorders, screening of the fetus. Chromatography and electrophoresis delineate patterns of amino-acid in urine and blood, and blood levels of amino-acids can now be measured. The normal newborn baby's urine has its own pattern of amino-acid excretion altered by the character of the milk feed and by drugs. Blood levels can only be interpreted correctly through knowledge of transport mechanisms as well as of ability to excrete and reabsorb amino-acids. Patients available for thorough study of all the many possible mechanisms have been too few for final answers to be given. Differences in the basic defect, which are associated with similar abnormalities in plasma and urine levels, may be responsible for differences in the clinical picture. It is not surprising that differences of interpretation persist.

Population studies have not yet provided final figures for neonatal incidence, but enough is known to show that, important as they are, all are rare conditions. To produce ten new patients with a particular disease in England and Wales in one year would require an incidence of the order of 1 in 80 000 live births. Incidence and management and cost are discussed in Chapter 18. The parents, or at least the mother, should be informed of the proposed tests and should be given the opportunity to refuse.

While the collection of blood and/or urine is the duty of nursing staff or of pathology technicians, it is essential that a doctor should be aware of what is happening, especially of the conditions under which the test is conducted. He should make plans to inform the parents of the test result even when this is negative.

Amniocentesis

Screening programmes depend on the availability of amniocentesis. This is valuable for the assessment in some cases of Rhesus iso-immunization, the assessment of fetal maturity, the likelihood of the respiratory distress syndrome and the pre-natal diagnosis of congenital and inherited conditions. The collection of 5–10 ml of fluid at the 14th week allows 3 weeks for cell culture and the possibility of termination of pregnancy at the 18th week.

In 1971 Rhesus iso-immunization caused a considerable morbidity and mortality, occupying a substantial amount of paediatric time in neonatal units. Inpatient spells for affected babies in 1971 (HIPE) numbered 2801 and there were 196 deaths. Stillbirths attributed to haemolytic disease of the newborn amounted to 338, another 187 dying within the first week of life. The general practitioner is concerned to identify women at risk and to ensure their delivery only in hospitals in which laboratory assessment before and after delivery and exchange transfusions can be competently managed. Only 12 consultations for haemolytic disease of the newborn are recorded for the 118 doctors in GPR. The present preventive treatment of rhesus-negative primiparous women is expected greatly to reduce the number who become immunized.

More accurate assessment of fetal maturity, too, should lessen the need for emergency special neonatal care, by bringing the situation under more accurate control. The lecithin/sphingomyelin ratio in amniotic fluid provides a measure of the risk of respiratory distress when induction of labour is being considered. The manpower and medical time required will be transferred from the paediatric staff to the obstetric and laboratory staff, but will not directly influence the work of the general practitioner.

The prenatal diagnosis of congenital and inherited conditions in the fetus should bring a reduction in the numbers of disabled and handicapped children. Quantification is difficult. Required are not only adequate facilities, but a general agreement about the wisdom and the ethics of a whole new set of indications for termination of pregnancy. Total prevention is not yet in sight and if it be the aim, this is bound to include the sacrifice of some normal fetuses. Application of present knowledge and techniques would certainly reduce the number of abnormal babies in the future. The most recent advance in measuring alpha-fetoprotein in amniotic fluid and in blood as a means of predicting anencephaly and the most severe forms of spina bifida (Brock *et al.* 1972) are referred to in Chapter 9. Out of a total of 3524 stillbirths and deaths in the first week from congenital anomalies, 1419 were anencephalic. Spina bifida and hydrocephalus accounted for another 768.

Chromosomal studies

The number of mongol babies could certainly be influenced by the study of cells from amniotic fluid. The present estimate is that 2.5 per cent of pregnancies in England and Wales occur in women over 40 years of age. They produce just under 20 per cent of the estimated 2000 or more annual births of mongols. At the age of over 35 years, the women responsible for 11 per cent of pregnancies produce 45 per cent of mongols. Translated into estimated numbers for 1971, the 20 000 mothers over 40 years produced 405 mongols and the 87 200 mothers aged over 35 years produced 909 mongols. Successful amniocentesis prediction to cut almost by half the annual intake of mongol babies into the population would require fluid examination for some 87 000 pregnant women, and the termination of pregnancy for some 900. Amniocentesis and the demonstration of normal chromosome structure can be used to avoid termination or grave maternal anxiety when there is a high risk of a second mongol birth.

Two other disabling conditions, haemophilia and classical pseudohypertrophic muscular dystrophy, could be reduced in numbers by establishing the male sex of the fetus in families where the disease is known. With present limited techniques, this would include the sacrifice of normal fetuses. There is no certain knowledge of the prevalence of these conditions in the child population and mutation muscular dystrophy (one third of the total) would not be prevented.

Prediction may be possible in time for cystic fibrosis. Certain inborn errors of metabolism and forms of lipo-chondrodystrophy are also expected to become predictable by amniocentesis. A campaign of preventive termination would reduce the numbers of affected children.

Without these methods the prevalence in the population of those conditions, which can be successfully treated with survival into adult life without infertility, is likely to increase.

Genetic counselling

There are now 28 general genetic clinics including one at each University Medical Centre. In addition there is one specialist clinic for each of the following, dermatology, ophthalmology and psychiatry.*

The general practitioner should be able to answer many of the questions, but if not he can refer to the appropriate specialist clinic or directly to a genetic clinic. This clinic would send the opinion on risk to the general practitioner, with whom the family should continue discussion.

As knowledge increases at the periphery, the functions of the central genetic clinic will change, but their main contribution will remain diagnosis when special cytogenetic or biochemical tests are needed or the carrying out of very complex calculations.

Genetic counselling is not free from the results of the general proposition that supply creates demand. Part of the clinic's work, for which allowance must be made, is bound to be to assist parents, prospective parents and families who consult for inappropriate reasons. While the reasons may be scientifically unsound, to free patients from anxieties, including unjustifiable ones, forms an essential part of a health service.

CARE OF THE INFANT AND THE PRE-SCHOOL CHILD

Routine surveillance of the normal baby

The later surveillance of the new baby is to be conducted through the Child Health Centre in conjunction with the general practitioner.

The movement towards the establishment of Infant Welfare Centres, now to be known as Child Health Centres, dates only from the end of the last century, although attempts had been made in previous centuries to carry out some of the functions. These included the instruction of mothers in infant feeding, the encouragement of breast feeding and the provision of sterilized cow's milk when breast milk was unavailable. The background to these endeavours was the prevention of gastroenteritis which took its annual toll of thousands of babies' lives. The

*'Human Genetics'. Prepared by The Standing Medical Advisory Committee for the Central Health Services Council and the Minister of Health 1972.

emphasis was therefore on elementary home hygiene and advice about feeding and milk formulae.

During the last fifty years the Health Visitor has played an increasing part both in health education and in giving detailed advice about care, hygiene and feeding. At the same time the doctor, freed from the original concern with gastro-enteritis, found himself more and more involved in advising about the management of the common behaviour disturbances presented by infants and toddlers, especially appetite, sleep and bowel problems. It seemed as if the spirit in which the bottle was given was at least as important as what was in it. Then two other major tasks arose: immunization against common communicable diseases began with diphtheria in the mid-thirties (see Chapter 15) and the total assessment of the child on the lookout for hidden handicaps started in a small way through the work of Dr Mary Sheridan with simple tests of hearing.

By 1964 the then Ministry of Health posed the question whether 'the centres are now needed for quite the same type of medical work as they were when they were first started . . .'. The Sheldon Committee was set up to provide the answers.

The recommendations (Sheldon 1967) for the functions of what were now to be called Child Health Centres were as follows:

1 Routine medical examinations of babies presumed healthy.
2 Infant nutrition and hygiene.
3 Appropriate care for immigrants with different culture and language problems.
4 Detection of defects, physical, mental and emotional.
5 Parent counselling over family problems.
6 Health education with particular reference to attitude towards training and behaviour.
7 Measurements of height (length) and weight.
8 Immunization on a prepared programme.
9 The sale of welfare and proprietary foods.

Changes since Sheldon

The Sheldon Committee's terms of reference being to review medical staffing and medical functions, the report dealt with the doctor, including the general practitioner, and the health visitor with only a mention of the importance of the patient's family and social background. Since 1967 attitudes and practices have changed in many ways. The reorganization of the social services has linked the hospital social services with those of the local authority although the methods of working of the two groups differ widely. At least three separate social workers, the health visitor, out patient and in-patient nursing staff, the midwife, and two or three different kinds of doctor may be involved in the preparation of the pregnant woman for her confinement, her actual confinement, the care of her newborn baby and its later surveillance. The teaching of the patient may suffer, as the result, at least from lack of continuity if not from inconsistency. The general practitioner with his 'attached' health visitor could provide both continuity and consistency.

Family planning by contraception and failed family planning with consequent counselling with a view to termination of pregnancy commonly introduce women to the first steps in taking or refusing responsibility for the outcome of sexual intercourse. Concurrence in proceeding with a pregnancy leads to antenatal care and preparation for labour and for the feeding and care of the baby. The pregnant woman's health, occupation, diet, smoking habits or other possible addictions are not the only matters to come under review. Her attitude and, when relevant, that of the father to the idea of parenthood and to breast feeding are also important.

A greater safety against death in infancy from gastro-enteritis used to be claimed correctly for breast feeding. There are now beginning to be important arguments, scientifically based in relation to immunology, against cow's milk feeding at least in the early weeks. A more positive encouragement of breast feeding is therefore justifiable. Opportunities should exist for the frank discussion of all these matters.

In the lying-in ward account must be taken of the importance of emotional bonding between mother and baby and the dangers of separation, while the emotional disturbance of the first few post-partum weeks with its moodiness and depression must be accepted and handled wisely by all attending staff.

Methods are now being studied through which families who are liable to get into difficulties with child rearing could be singled out. Ideally special steps should be taken to support and advise them during the early days after mother and baby go home. A concentration of effort on these families at this period might be a critical contribution to family health not only through ensuring a more successful breast feeding but also in establishing good relationships within the family. Somewhat less attention paid to successfully developing families would not be too high a price to pay.

Unfortunately from the mother's point of view many different systems are supported by the professionals for feeding, weaning on to solids, so-called sphincter training, discipline, and even immunization against infectious disease. Whatever the details, and no-one can properly claim that all methods but his own are wrong, the long-term aim should be to train mothers to make their own decisions, going the way of their own grain, so that after the next pregnancy they can manage most of the routines themselves. Some incompetent, unteachable and unreliable mothers will always remain to provide a target for health and social services.

Immunization is undertaken in the Child Health Centre. Early referral for assessment of speech problems, and of hearing and sight including squints are referred to in Chapter 6. Information about the common causes of accidents, especially in the home, about prevention and the best steps when they do occur can well be given at this time (see Chapter 19). The special problems of immigrant children are discussed in Chapter 21 and of stressful family situations in Chapter 20.

Two further questions await answers—what place the Child Health Centre should occupy in under- and post-graduate training, and how to supervise the important group of non-attenders for whom such supervision may be of paramount importance.

Babies 'at risk'

Butler has shown in the 1958 cohort that leaving aside what was observable at birth, certain circumstances increased the liability to hidden handicaps. These include maternal rubella, low birth weight (below 4.5 lb, 2.5 kg), severe perinatal hypoxia, hyperbilirubinaemia, advancing birth order and sibship of genetically determined disorders. The incidence was higher among the offspring of unskilled workers. For prevention, the effective factor or factors need to be identified, for example, is it overcrowding, bad housing, poor physical conditions, or is it incompetence from a low intelligence or inadequate personality with failure to manage life's problems or stresses? The probability that several factors are involved has to be remembered.

Knox and Mahon (1970), linking maternity data with the likelihood of a need for special education at age 13 years, were able to implicate low birth weight, traumatic delivery and the indices of social underprivilege. Nevertheless, they concluded that as practised the 'at risk' Register has not justified its existence. Alberman and Goldstein (1970) using National Child Development Study data have examined the joint effects of certain predictors of handicap and have argued against the complete abandonment of the 'at risk' concept. Taking the adverse risks as parity 4 or more, abnormal delivery by an untrained person and illness in the baby's first week of life, they showed that this combination did present a valuable predictor and they concluded that babies subjected to these risks deserved to be examined more frequently than the 'normal' population, perhaps four times as often. It may be that the surveillance of such babies should be the responsibility of the most experienced paediatricians in the locality.

The hidden handicaps include congenital malformations involving internal organs, especially the cardiovascular system, and hipjoints, defects of vision, and some metabolic disorders. The benefit of early identification may be to minimize the resulting disability. The most difficult and the most worrying are neuropsychiatric disorders. The presence of gross neurological disorders and mental handicap should become apparent during the first year.

Bearing these possibilities in mind, the further routine medical examinations recommended by Sheldon are at 6 months, with a hearing test at each birthday, one, two, three and four. The cover test for squint should also be undertaken. Hearing and squint tests should be repeated at 3- and 4-year-old examination with a dental examination. Visual acuity should be tested at the fourth birthday, and there may later be screening tests for the possibility of learning handicap.

Developmental assessment is already carried out by good community doctors and some general practitioners in many parts of the country. This periodic assessment of the whole child takes into account motor, sensory, language, performance and social skills as well as the child's behaviour, ability to concentrate and to make relationships. A five-man practice with 20 000 to 25 000 patients would include 1500 children under the age of five years. Dr Curtis Jenkins (1973) estimates that two doctors doing two half-day sessions each week would be able to carry out adequate assessments, each lasting 15 minutes, on pre-school children. He allows for three examinations during the first year, two in the second and an annual one at three and four years.

During the last ten years 75 to 80 assessment centres have been established through the country staffed by multi-disciplinary teams and linked with community health services. Teaching courses in the required techniques have been developed at the Wolfson Centre and the Newcomen Clinic in London. Others are run by the Society of Community Medicine and by some university departments and the subject is properly included in vocational courses for general practitioners.

The pre-school child is attracting sociological interest. As far as doctors are concerned, the reticence of the toddler, his sudden unfriendliness after his first birthday that replaces his earlier happy smiles of greeting, has been respected to the detriment of medical knowledge. The limits of normal behaviour are wide, the rate of progress variable, or so it is believed. While it is true that the new baby's personality is recognizable at birth or shortly after, characteristics that shape patterns of behaviour seem established by the age of five years. Questions that may be of life-long importance cannot always be answered. What has been happening during these three or four years? Is it correct that variation is wide and that the extremes have no significance? The temper tantrums, the aggression, the food refusal, the persistent incontinence, should they be regarded as 'within the normal limits' or are these cries for help in a language that is misunderstood? The baby in the first year and the schoolchild throughout receive detailed attention. Perhaps the time has come for special studies of the health and behaviour of the children in between.

CHAPTER 4

Growth and its disorders

Child health ensures an optimal rate of growth. The assumption is that for every child such an optimal rate exists and that periodic assessment of the child is desirable until growth ceases. Certainly those concerned with child health needs must be aware of the factors, genetic, environmental and morbid which may contribute to deviation from the optimal. Traditionally physical growth, the simplest to measure, has been the main object of both parental interest and scientific study. More recently intellectual growth has been subjected to assessment, although the validity of different methods remains controversial. Most recently of all, efforts have been made to measure emotional adjustment by comparing maturation of habit and behaviour with anticipated normals.

Many studies have contributed to the understanding of the close relationships between bodily growth, educational success and emotional adjustment. Twenty-five years ago, Widdowson (1948) in an article on 'Mental contentment and physical growth' concluded that 'psychological stresses due to harsh and unsympathetic handling may seriously curtail growth rates'. She had carefully measured the differences in growth rates of children on fixed diets in two orphanages, one being in the charge of a lady who ruled with a rod of iron, but had favourites and who, by good fortune for the study, transferred with her favourites to the previously happy orphanage in the course of the observations. The moral for Widdowson was that 'even the most perfectly planned nutritional investigation may be ruined by factors over which the investigator may have no control'. The moral for the paediatrician arises from his knowledge that emotional factors must be remembered both in the planning of observations and in the interpretation of results. And it provides an objective basis for the use of records of physical growth in the assessment of emotional well-being.

The availability of methods of estimating human growth hormone have begun to transform a somewhat mystical and previously mysterious connexion between happiness and bodily growth into hard scientific data. The simulation of idiopathic hypopituitarism by the effects of emotional deprivation was noted by Powell *et al.* (1967 a, b) in observations on 13 children, whose growth accelerated markedly when they were removed from deprived family life to a convalescent home. The home background included marital stress, promiscuity, alcoholism and immaturity of parents. Apart from retarded growth the children showed polydipsia, bizarre drinking and eating habits, coeliac-like syndrome and actual food deprivation. In two families there were non-accidental injuries. Hormone studies revealed deficiency of ACTH and of growth hormone release.

Similar effects on pituitary function were demonstrated by Krieger and Mellinger (1971) in children whose dwarfism resulted from nutritional deprivation and also in emotionally deprived 'psycho-social dwarfism'.

The interaction between emotional stress, appetite and food intake is all too apparent to the doctor in his work with children who won't eat or who eat too much.

Both dwarfism and gigantism affect school achievement. Pollitt and Money (1964) have shown that while intelligence as measured is not itself affected, dwarf children underfunction in school. 'The challenge of being a member of a group appears to be more important to them than their school work.' Just as children of large stature tend to be treated even by their parents as older than their calendar or mental age, so small children tend to be 'babied'. Notoriety at school is inevitable and may be greeted by the child either with mortification or with delight in the resulting popularity. Pollitt and Money point out that when hormone therapy succeeds in removing the special status of the dwarf, his need for a considerable emotional adjustment must be met with understanding by teachers and parents. The reaction may be sufficiently severe for further treatment to be rejected by the patient, for whom psychotherapy might then be needed.

The process of assessment begins with the examination of the newborn baby, referred to in Chapter 3, continues in the Child Health Clinic with developmental assessments as well as periodic weighing. When the child enters school the medical interest in repeated assessment usually comes to an end, unless special attention is drawn to the child by reason of illness, educational failure, parental anxiety or some general observation by school teacher or educational welfare officer.

Whether the continuation of specialized interest during school years with all the expense of skilled personnel and time can be justified is arguable. The general practitioner should be able to attempt periodic assessment, were he so minded, when he sees the child for some acute incident. Something more than that the child 'looks alright' and 'seems to be getting along well enough' might be necessary. The use of growth charts, even if not of the ultimate sophistication of those devised by

Tanner (Tanner *et al.* 1970), would at least serve as a screening method. Opportunity could also be taken to ask a few questions about school progress and maturation of habit and behaviour.

Towards the end of childhood, problems may arise connected with onset of puberty. Parental anxiety may centre around the development of genitalia, the quantity or distribution of hair, and the appearance of breast tissue in girls especially when one breast appears before the other. The effects of puberty development on emotional adjustment, intra-familial relationships, and attitudes to education, careers and sexual behaviour are better recognized than understood. The foundations for these problems may well have been laid during earlier years. Nevertheless, late thought it may be, the cost to society in wasted talents, legal processes and damage to property besides ruined health, and social and moral dilemmas over illegitimate births and pregnancy termination may justify specialization by doctors and social workers in the age period of adolescence. *Finis coronat opus.* The care and concern about the needs of child health during earlier years is largely wasted if it fails to ensure that the young adult is fitted to take the responsible part both in society and in his own family life which his skills and aptitudes allow.

The obvious association between disease processes and disordered growth is now more widely appreciated by parents and teachers as well as by doctors. The child's emotional reaction to his size is not always taken into account in the management of children with such growth retarding conditions as cyanotic congenital heart disease, chronic renal failure, severe chronic anaemia, such as occurs in thalassaemia when haemoglobin is not maintained above 8 g per 100 ml (Kattamis *et al.* 1970). Nor is it easy to discern when a child whose growth remains well within the range of normal is in reality not following his 'correct' growth curve. The steady increase in absolute heights of child populations when socio-economic conditions improve illustrates this point.

The list taken from Parkin (1972–73) contains the main headings for the common causes of disordered growth (Table 4.1). There is no information about the prevalence of growth problems. In the Newcastle Community Study, a sample of 82 'short normal children' was investigated. The mothers had sought medical advice from either the family doctor or the school medical officer in only 8, although the mother was worried in another 11, yet took no action. In 57 out of 82 no anxiety was expressed (Parkin 1975).

What is suggested here is that the periodic assessment of the growth of children provides one of the most valuable indices of total child health.

Table 4.1. Classification of some commoner causes of disordered growth
(From Parkin 1972-73)

Group	*Short stature*	*Tall stature*
Genetic	Familial short stature	Familial tall stature
Intra-uterine	Placental insufficiency Infections of fetus	
Nutritional	Inadequate food supply Infections Malabsorption	Simple obesity
Systemic disease	Congenital cardiac disease Chronic renal disease Disorder of central nervous system	
Bone diseases	Congenital, e.g. achondroplasia Acquired, e.g. rickets	
Specific syndromes (chromosomal and others)	Turner's syndrome Silver's syndrome	XYY karyotype Cerebral gigantism
Endocrine	Growth hormone deficiency Thyroid deficiency Corticosteroid excess Precocious puberty or pseudo-precocious puberty	Growth hormone excess Thyroid excess Precocious puberty and pseudo-precocious puberty
Emotional	Deprivation	
Variation in development	Delayed growth or puberty	Early puberty

Disorders of appetite, obesity

The central position occupied by feeding during the first two or three years of life is well appreciated by all who are concerned with infant care. The mother's feeling of responsibility is intense both about the quantity and the quality of the food given and received. Even the young baby quickly realizes the strength of the influence which his meal-time behaviour has upon his mother's emotions. The mother's lap or the high chair at feeding times provides one battlefield for the conflict between mother's domination and baby's independence or even the baby's domination with roles reversed. The doctor finds so often that the tension at meal times is the key to other behaviour disturbances and that, if with time the tension has been allowed to grow, relief is very difficult to obtain.

At a superficial level this is a matter for education and instruction and should play an important part in health education. At a deeper level, cultural patterns and apparently innate prejudices strongly influence the mother's reactions. At an even deeper level, basic instinctive relationships between individuals, baby, mother and at times mother and grandmother play their part, with father in the wings.

In a deprived society inadequate feeding, with its effect in limiting growth, depends upon scarcity. As a society develops, this aspect is disregarded and inadequate provision of food usually results from family incompetence. The Child Health Clinic and the Health Visitor have the responsibility for identifying such problems and for taking appropriate steps to overcome the difficulties. In the affluent society material scarcity is replaced by emotional surfeit.

The part played by the doctor is important, although less important than it was since the training of midwives and health visitors has given them the right to a more authoritarian voice. Unfortunately food fads are not confined to children and many adults, including the doctors, have theories and practices which are the more strongly held the less are their scientific foundation. Hence repeated changes in the recommendations, for example for high calorie feeding, for the time and the order for beginning solids, for the need for routine or for 'on demand' feeding of babies.

Two conditions, one common and one rare, exhibit extremes of appetite disorder, for which medical advice is usually sought, obesity and anorexia nervosa. As usual, study of extremes has a fascination seldom excited by run-of-the-mill problems, and, as usual, the information gleaned has a wider application. The first systematic study of obese children was undertaken by Bruch (1939–40) and her work established beyond dispute the existence of psycho-social factors. Some specific neurological and endocrinological diseases are associated with obesity, but in most types of human obesity 'there is probably an interrelationship between psycho-social, biochemical, neurophysiological and hereditary processes' (Glucksman 1972). It is not surprising that long-term observations on obese children treated by diet restriction alone are disappointing (Lloyd *et al.* 1961). Hospital admission is usually unnecessary and the estimate in HIPE is 697, all but 22 in the 5- to 14-year-old group. GPR counted 202 in this age group in the sample, 136 in girls with a consultation rate of 5.8 per 1000 population. This represents an important and time consuming element in practice. A review of 400 recent references to treatment by Penick and Stunkard (1972) failed to show more than a modest improvement in results, to which drugs and hormones have not contributed. Fasting, group treatments, behaviour modification for individuals and groups, and patient self-help groups appear to have been of real value in the management of obese women. These methods do not seem applicable to children. The problem is large enough and of long enough duration to call for detailed study on a co-operative basis.

No particular attention appears to have been paid to prevention. Heald (1972) concludes that no direct relationship exists between birth weight and obesity (defined as 20 per cent or more above expected weight). A better predictor is the rate of weight gain in the first six months (Eid 1970). The fear of an excessive weight gain has in the past influenced mothers to limit the baby's food even at the price of his happiness. More recently high calorie feeding has been fashionable but now anxiety about the effect on cholesterol levels in the blood has swung the pendulum in the other direction.

Many mothers seek medical advice about feeding their babies especially the first born. Unfortunately this need can only be met by the doctor with dogmatism and inevitably the doctor tends to develop a stereotyped system. In consultation he lacks the time to present the principles from which his system is derived. The gaps in current knowledge need to be filled, not only so that advice may be soundly based but also because the interaction between mother and baby over meals often sets its particular seal on their future relationship. This is an important child health need for research as well as for teaching. The need cannot be quantified. Suffice it to say that a review of feeding methods and their success forms part of every consultation about a baby and should form part of at least the first consultation of every child over the age of two years. The influence which the health visitor and the nurse in charge of the maternity unit may have upon feeding patterns must never be ignored.

CHAPTER 5

Malformations

All malformations are important. How important depends on the view point of the person making the judgement. The doctor has his own priorities headed by malformations that are lethal, and among these the main challenge is to recognize at the earliest moment those that are treatable. Next in importance is interference with function, either primary, from the malformation itself or secondary, because the defect interferes with some other organ or system or with development of one or other skills. Probably at the bottom of his list are malformations which have only a cosmetic influence. On the other hand for the patient and his family the cosmetic malformation may prove the hardest of all to bear and much time-consuming support and consolation may be needed from the doctor. A large facial naevus or a hemivertebra causing scoliosis and torticollis are serious in that while they do not greatly disturb physical function they may interfere with social function and distort the development of character and personality. Plastic surgeons have learnt from burned patients the harmful and pervasive effects of disfigurement on self-esteem. Children and their parents are not immune from these dangers.

Quantification of the incidence of malformations detectable at birth has been attempted through a scheme of notification operated since 1964 by the Department of Health and the General Register Office. The main object, following the thalidomide tragedy, is to recognize early by means of monthly computer studies any significant change in one or more of eighty malformations selected mainly because they are easy to recognize. Table 5.1 shows the nine sub-headings under which the individual malformations are grouped.

The pattern remains relatively consistent from 1969 to 1973, malformations of the limbs contributing about 40 per cent, those of the central nervous system about 25 per cent, cleft lip and/or cleft palate 8 per cent and malformation of the external genitalia 7 per cent. These figures have only a limited value in relation to treatment needs. Diagnosis in the early days of life is inevitably inaccurate. For example hearing a heart murmur is not the same as diagnosing a malformation. The murmur may disappear while a serious cardiac malformation may not reveal its presence until much later. Accessory auricles are easily

Table 5.1. Congenital malformations notified at birth
(Numbers of babies born with each malformation by type of birth, 1971, with totals for 1972 and 1973: and rates for each malformation per 10 000 total births for 1971, 1972 and 1973. GRO figures)

SITE	*Numbers of malformations*		*TOTALS (include incomplete records)*			*Rate per 10 000 total babies*		
	Live	Still	1971	1972	1973	1971	1972	1973
All babies	12 534	1 812	14 407	14 412	13 353	182.0	196.3	195.3
Central nervous system	1 863	1 496	3 378	3 129	2 553	42.6	42.6	37.3
Eye	98	9	107	138	99	1.3	1.9	1.4
Ear	384	8	393	413	393	5.0	5.6	5.7
Cleft lip and/or palate	989	72	1 063	997	985	13.4	13.6	14.4
Intestines	499	26	532	497	448	6.7	6.8	6.6
Cardiovascular system	696	16	714	803	725	9.0	10.9	10.6
External genitalia	1 115	16	1 136	1 182	1 125	14.3	16.1	16.4
Limbs	5 033	158	5 206	5 116	4 611	65.6	69.7	67.4
Chromosomes	601	30	632	615	571	8.0	8.4	8.3

recognized while a pre-auricular sinus is probably ignored more often than noted and neither is of any real significance. Among the urogenital system malformations feature hydrocele and undescended testicle. Hydroceles are common enough to be regarded in many cases as variations of the normal and often resolve spontaneously; the status of a diagnosis of undescended testicle within the early days of life is questionable to say the least. These figures are of potential value for their stated purpose namely to show some sudden change in frequency or pattern which might lead to the early recognition and consequent withdrawal of a new iatrogenic drug. That they fail to provide a valid index of the incidence of congenital malformations in the population is not surprising since this was not their original intention.

Another approach may be made through a study of HIPE and RGSR (1971) in class XIV of which congenital anomalies are listed. For any accurate estimate of the toll in morbidity and mortality of congenital anomalies, these tables are as unsuitable as the table recording notifications of congenital malformations recognized at birth. The absence from

Classes of congenital malformation notified on GRO Form SD. 56

Central nervous system	Urino-genital system
Eye and ear	Limbs
Alimentary system	Other parts of musculo-skeletal system
Heart and circulatory system	Other systems
Respiratory system	Other malformations

this class of diaphragmatic hernia which caused 89 deaths in the first week of life and the presence of undescended testes, 10 763, and congenital dislocation of the hip, 3422, with presumably no deaths, that is to say the impossibility of considering the lethal or potentially lethal separately from the non-lethal, prevents the use of the data for valid conclusions about illness and death resulting from congenital anomalies as a whole. Nevertheless some practical points arise to which attention is drawn.

There were 60 858 discharges and deaths in these 20 groups (ICD 740–759). They are shown in Table 5.2 with the total number of childhood deaths from RGSR Table 17, and the deaths under one month of age are listed separately. Of the 3627 deaths, 19.7 per cent occurred on the first day, 38.6 per cent within the first week, 55 per cent during the first month and 81 per cent during the first year of life. The discharges and

Table 5.2. Class XIV congenital anomalies

ICD No.		HIPE 1971	RGSR 1971 deaths 1st month	0–14 yrs	Remarks
740	Anencephalus	33	163	169	1054 deaths = 29.0 per cent of total deaths. 69 per cent result from spina bifida and hydrocephalus (740–743)
741	Spina bifida	4 540	371	608	
742	Congenital hydrocephalus	1 362	50	121	
743	Other congenital anomalies of nervous system	775	75	156	
	Congenital anomalies				
744	of eye	2 159	1	1	
745	of ear, face and neck	3 510	3	3	
746	of heart	6 170	615	1 472	1665 deaths = 45.9 per cent of total deaths: of these, 43 per cent in first month and 75 per cent in first year (746–747)
747	others of circulatory system	1 838	104	193	
748	of respiratory tract	1 096	73	85	
749	cleft palate and hare lip	2 757	6	12	
750	others of upper alimentary tract	3 776	43	60	
751	others of digestive system	1 993	73	170	
752	of genital organs	13 852	1	2	
753	of urinary system	930	114	154	
754	club foot (congenital)	4 241	4	4	
755	others of limbs	7 009	6	9	
756	others of musculo-skeletal system	1 916	54	73	
757	of skin, hair and nails	1 141	5	9	
758	other and unspecified	775	27	46	
759	multiple systems	985	209	280	
	Total	60 858	1 997	3 627	

deaths after the first week of life numbered 52 459. Between the ages of one and fifteen years there were 577 deaths 65 per cent of which were due to congenital disease of heart and circulatory system.

The *nervous system* lesions (ICD 740–3) contribute 6704 to the HIPE total (7.3 per cent) and their mean stay in hospital is among the longest.

Spina bifida is discussed in Chapter 9 and the involvement of many specialists in hospital and in out-patients is great. Antenatal identification if followed by pregnancy termination would therefore relieve the Health Service of a great deal of work.

The anomalies of *heart and circulatory system* contribute 7975 to the HIPE total (8.7 per cent). 104 deaths on the first day and a further 331 by the end of the first week, total 435, 27 per cent of deaths in these groups and 12.2 per cent of all the childhood deaths in class XIV. A fuller discussion of implications will be found in Chapter 16.

Anomalies of the *respiratory tract* (ICD 748) numbered 1096 with 85 deaths, 69 during the first week. Of 2757 cleft palate and hare lip discharges (ICD 749) with 12 deaths, 1229 related to the first year and 908 to from one to four years, 77.5 per cent of the discharges occurring below the age of five years. The incidence of cleft palate alone is calculated as 1:2500 and of cleft lip and palate as 1:500. These estimates would suggest, for 1971, 313 of the former and 1566 of the latter making a total of 1879 fresh cases for treatment compared with 1229 discharges and deaths under one year. The children were presumably admitted for plastic surgery. The mean duration of stay for this age group was between 10 and 20 days, an average of 40 admitted each week. Joint arrangements between plastic surgical and paediatric units are required. These have caused difficulty in the past, the plastic surgical units being often located in hospitals lacking paediatric services.

For the other congenital anomalies of the *upper alimentary tract* and of the *digestive system* (ICD 750–1), the prime requirement is skilled diagnosis. Nearly all are treatable, so that expert surgery, anaesthesia and nursing should be available. The outlook, however, is greatly worsened when there are additional serious defects and when delay in treatment leads to dangerous or lethal complications. Taking the two groups together, the HIPE total is 5769 (6.3 per cent) with 230 deaths, 72 (31 per cent) in the first week.

Pyloric stenosis with an incidence of 1:150 boys and 1:775 girls, should have occurred in 3178 babies. HIPE does not provide a separate heading. One death is recorded in the second year of life.

Other lesions of the digestive tract (ICD 751) were responsible for 1993 discharges and deaths. Two important conditions are notoriously difficult to treat, tracheo-oesophageal fistula and Hirschsprung's disease causing 54 and 29 deaths respectively. Atresia of the small intestine, which should be treatable in the majority, caused 48 deaths, anomalies of intestinal fixation 9, atresia of the rectum and anal canal 12, and other intestinal anomalies 8. It is interesting to compare the actual number of reported deaths with the accepted incidence of conditions occurring in newborn babies. Live births in 1971 numbered 783 155. Tracheo-oesophageal fistula (1 : 3000) should have appeared 261 times; it caused 50 deaths in the first year. Of Hirschsprung's disease (1 : 25 000) there should have been 32 new cases RGSR reports 25 deaths in the first year. Atresia of the intestine (1 : 10 000) should have occurred in 78 new babies. All of the 48 reported deaths occurred before the eighth week except one which died between two and six months. Imperforate anus (1 : 5000) should have occurred in 156. This is sometimes missed at first but carries a good prognosis unless associated with considerable rectal atresia. Ten out of the twelve deaths occurred in the first six months.

All of these babies do need the services of a skilled neonatal surgical department, but this will not improve results in the general population without experienced and informed observation by midwives, obstetricians, paediatricians and general practitioners. Speed is of the essence. With oesophageal and high small intestine obstruction delay is especially dangerous and this is shown by the number of deaths in the first week, 30 out of 54 in tracheo-oesophageal fistula, 22 out of 48 in small intestine atresia, and 4 out of 9 with anomalies of fixation, a condition usually associated with duodenal obstruction.

Anomalies of the *gall bladder, liver and bile ducts* caused 49 deaths, 23 in the first year. These are seldom easily treatable.

Congenital anomalies of the genital organs provided 13 852 discharges, 25.7 per cent of the total, with only 2 deaths. Undescended testicle forms the major group with 10 763, which is 20 per cent of the whole class and 77.7 per cent of the genital anomalies. In the list of operations (HIPE Table 22i) orchidopexy was performed 9844 times, mainly in the 5 to 14 years group, An additional 2015 operations were performed on the testes and adnexa, which probably included many for congenital anomalies other than those recorded as 'undescended testicles'. In the urinary tract, a small group of 930, there was by contrast a high mortality with no less than 154 deaths, 135 within the first year, 92 within the first week. Renal agenesis has an incidence of 1 : 3500 and ectopia vesicae of 1 : 50 000. There should have been 224 of the former and 15 of the latter in the year. The disparity cannot be explained by failure to record some of those with renal agenesis as live births, since only 22 stillbirths are attributed to congenital anomalies of the genito-urinary system. RGSR singles out 34 deaths from cystic kidney disease, 31 within the first 9 weeks.

Orthopaedic anomalies include club foot (4241) and others of limbs

(7009). Together they provide 13 deaths, 8 on the first day. Presumably the actual cause of death must be sought elsewhere. Congenital dislocation of the hip numbers 3422 in the HIPE, 897 in the first year. An incidence of 1 : 15 000 would have produced 522 new cases. Unspecified other anomalies of the *musculo-skeletal system* (1916) contributed 73 deaths, 40 on the first day and 48 in the first week.

No comment is offered about the anomalies of *skin, hair and nails* or the *'other and unspecified anomalies'* (ICD 758). The last group of congenital syndromes affecting *multiple systems* numbered 985 discharges and deaths. There were 280 deaths, 209 of which occurred in the first month of life (74.6 per cent). 'Down's disease' is included in this group and accounted for 43 deaths.

Some additional data

A few special surveys of incidence and prevalence of malformations have been carried out. These have concerned relatively small populations and have had objectives varying from the purely statistical to attempting correlations with social class or some other particular. Or the relationship studied has been the practical one of social and environmental help required by reason of the severity of the resulting handicap. From none of these has it been possible to use the figures to illuminate the need for medical, surgical or other 'Health Service' attention. Prevalence figures are given in the chapters that deal with chronic handicaps of various kinds and with system and organ 'diseases'. There seems to be a general acceptance of an incidence rate for congenital malformations of about 25 per 1000 total birth. In 1971 this would have totalled a little less than 19 600.

Table 5.3 gives the results of two Birmingham surveys, the first (I) by McKeown and Record (1960) on 56 760 consecutive births, 1950 to 1952, and the second (II) by Lack (1964) on a total birth population of 147 500, 1957 to 1963. The former workers defined a malformation as a 'macroscopic abnormality of structure attributable to faulty development and present at birth'. They concentrated their study on eight structural defects and collected information at 2 weeks and again at 5 years by which age one half of the malformed children (4.3 per cent of the total births) had died. Lack listed twelve structural defects. The rates derived by Lack and McKeown's corrected 5-year rates have been applied to the 1971 births. Unfortunately the rates all relate to total live and still births so that the treatment and management needs for those born alive and, with a number of the conditions, those surviving the perinatal period cannot be counted.

Table 5.3. Birmingham Studies: malformations among consecutive births with 1971 projections

(Rates per 1000 births)

	I N=56 760 1950–52	II N=147 570 1957–63	*Projection of numbers* N=783 155 1971
Neural			
Anencephalus	1.96	2.26	1 535–1 770
Spina bifida	3.00	—	2 349
with cephalocele	—	2.62	2 052
Hydrocephalus	2.57	—	2 013
Mongol	1.69	—	1 323
Alimentary			
Cleft lip and palate	1.94	1.17	1 519–916
Cleft palate alone	—	0.61	478
Oesophageal atresia	—	0.34	266
Tracheo-oesophageal fistula			
Anal atresia	—	0.35	274
Exomphalos	—	0.44	344
Diaphragmatic (not hiatus) hernia	—	0.40	313
Limbs			
Talipes	4.44	—	3 477
Congenital dislocation of the hip	0.67	0.65*	525–509
Amelia, phocomelia	—	0.18	141
Defects of thumb and/or radii	—	0.13	102
Renal agenesis			
Urogenital	—	0.33	258
(bilateral)			
All with one or more of the above	—	8.35	6 539
All malformed individuals	23.08	—	18 075

* Live births only (Record and Edwards 1958)
I = McKeown and Record 1960
II = Lack 1964

CHAPTER 6

Disorders of vision, hearing, speech and communication

VISUAL HANDICAP

Visual defects and squint, actual or latent, are responsible for about one quarter of all the defects that need inspection in the school population. Franceschetti considers that 15 per cent of school children should be referred to an ophthalmologist (XX International Congress of Ophthalmology 1966), a figure consistent with the finding in the National Development Study that 14 per cent of school children had some defect of vision (NCB). Squint operations provide also an important reason for admission of children to hospital for surgical treatment. Screening tests for sight and for the presence of squint are routine procedures in general infant assessment, for all school entrants and periodically through the school surveillance.

Blind and partially sighted children

The Vernon Report (1972) accepted a prevalence in the school population in January 1971 of 1.37 per 10 000 blind (1207) and 2.66 per 10 000 partially sighted (2338), a total of 4.03 per 10 000 children (3545) aged 5 to 19 years in England and Wales. These figures do not accurately reveal population prevalence, but rather the prevalence of visual defect that has led to a need for special education. The children were attending schools for the partially sighted or special units attached to normal schools or schools for other handicaps. A few were awaiting admission.

An analysis in 1969 of 1916 partially sighted school children (see Table 6.1) showed that 449 (23 per cent) had another handicap affecting education, one third of whom were assessed as educationally subnormal. A further 423 children had an additional problem which complicated management although not requiring special educational treatment in its own right. Visual impairment and blindness are not always in the records of children with other severe handicaps.

The harmful effects of visual defects are exaggerated by the presence of any other form of deprivation. Often the visual defect is one among a number of congenital defects, including neurological and intellectual deficits. The 'normal blind' child is becoming a rarity.

Table 6.1. Serious defect in 449 children in 1969 in schools for partially sighted children or in units attached to ordinary or other special schools (Vernon 1972).

n = 1916

ESN	155	Hearing defect	18
Physically handicapped	47	Speech defect	31
Epilepsy	25	Speech defect and hearing defect	53
Maladjusted	25	Speech defect and low IQ	56
Delicate	9	Physically handicapped and low IQ	30

Table 6.2. Taken from Sorsby (1972) lists the percentage distribution of causes contributing more than 3.5 per cent of the total registration of 1963–68.

Cause	*Percentages* *Age*: 0–4	5–14 *years*
Congenital defect	70.0	54.1
Optic atrophy acquired or presumed acquired	9.9	19.3
Retrolental fibroplasia	6.3	4.1
Retinoblastoma	3.6	—
Retinitis pigmentosa	—	4.9
All other	10.2	17.6
Prevalence per 100 000 population	2.5	4.0

Sorsby (1972) has reviewed the incidence and causes of blindness in England and Wales for the years 1963–68 (Table 6.2). In 1968 out of a total registered blind population of 102 693 children aged 0–14 years accounted for 2133, including 267 newly registered, a prevalence of 22.2 per 10 000 with a rate of 2.4 per 10 000 newly registered during the year. Of those under 5 years old one quarter were totally blind compared with one tenth in the group 5–14 years. There had been little change in total numbers over the years. He suggested that better preventive treatment was being balanced by the increased survival of vulnerable newborn babies.

A sex difference, not apparent under 5 years, becomes marked later with males predominating (201 M to 164 F), especially among those with retinitis pigmentosa (21 M to 9 F). Patients with retrolental fibroplasia are still found, about 10 each year under the age of 5 years and 5 more during school life. A review of 224 children resident in Sunshine Homes (1963–68) of whom 41 were admitted in 1968, showed the main cause of blindness to be a congenital defect (114). The defects include cataract (33), microphthalmia (18) and retinal abnormalities (16). Retrolental fibroplasia was present in 21, undetermined optic atrophy in 64, and visual impairment was caused by infection in 9 and by fetal rubella in 7. Educational and management problems of the greatest difficulty are presented by the 'blind-deaf' children of whom 206 under the age of 6 years were known to principal school medical officers in January 1968.

Children with visual handicap are found frequently among the mentally handicapped and about one third of all blind children are deemed ineducable, which is another way of saying that methods suitable for their education are not yet available. There is a serious lack of education services even for those educable children whose parents refuse residential schooling for them.

Many affected children and their families are seriously emotionally disturbed, giving importance to parent counselling from the time of diagnosis. Dr Shirley Fine (1968) concluded that these children were more liable to emotional disturbance than sighted children. This has not been confirmed in studies in which a more generous view is taken of the level of emotional disturbance in sighted children.

In January 1971 there were 18 special schools for the blind and 19 for the partially sighted with 256 on the roll. Adolescents could receive further education in three establishments.

Assessment teams

The Vernon Report recommends that assessment should be a team project and that the team should include, besides the ophthalmologist, a paediatrician, a local authority medical officer, a general practitioner, an otologist, a health visitor and a social worker. To this might be added a psychologist with special experience. The omission of an orthoptist is curious in relation to the size of the squint problem. This team should work in the school setting. No estimate is given of the number of such teams, but an annual test of visual acuity is advised.

Genetic counselling

Dr Fine (1968) has stressed the importance of genetic counselling since a genetic aetiology may be present in as many as 40 per cent. This is especially needed in families in which retinoblastoma is found.

Squint

The 1958 Cohort study at 7 years showed the presence of a squint in 3.5 per cent (NCB). In 43 per cent of these children the vision even of the better eye was impaired. A past squint had been suspected or reported in a further 3.9 per cent. Alberman, Butler and Gardiner (1971) have shown that cerebral palsy, mental subnormality or clumsiness were twice as common in children with squints as in a control group and that poor speech, left or mixed handedness and signs of maladjustment were significantly increased. Their findings also confirmed the earlier discovery by the Newcastle observers (Miller *et al.* 1960) of a higher incidence of squint among the children who fulfilled their criteria of deficient care. Further, even when clumsy children and those suspected of mild cerebral dysfunction were excluded, a disproportionate number of poor readers remained. While it is agreed that all babies with squints should be examined by ophthalmologists and orthoptists before the age of one year, the correlations that have been established strongly support the need for a much closer liaison throughout childhood between ophthalmologists, orthoptists and paediatricians than usually exists now, a viewpoint strengthened by the 1968 Symposium on Developmental and Paediatric Ophthalmology (Clinics in Developmental Medicine, No. 32).

The average number of squint operations for 100 000 population (HIPE 1971) is given as:

	Males	*Females*
Aged 0 to 4 years	299.2	287.4
Aged 5 to 14 years	180.5	174.1

Preventive treatment

The number of children with squint amblyopia leading to permanent deterioration of visual acuity in the suppressed eye should be reduced if all squints were recognized before the first birthday and adequately treated.

The HIPE estimate is that of the 25 269 operations on the muscles of the eyeball in children under the age of 15 years, over half (54.5 per cent) were performed on children over the age of 5 years and therefore late by standard practice. Although the mean duration of stay in hospital is only four days, the need to perform this operation is a major cause for the admission of children to hospital. Would any form of preventive action cut down this requirement and at the same time prevent the amblyopia? Screening tests of hearing acuity have been firmly introduced into the assessment of infants, and, although not always accurately performed, have contributed to better treatment. A similar urgency does not seem to have been imparted to the assessment of visual acuity and especially to the detection of failure of development of co-ordinated binocular vision. Many ophthalmologists consider that an orthoptist would be the best person to make the earliest diagnosis of strabismus. Despite the recommended screening in the child health clinic at 1, 2 and 3 years, the number of children needing operations does not fall. An important present child health need is easy access to an orthoptist for any baby showing suspicious signs of squint to be followed by referral to an ophthalmologist with a view to exercises under orthoptist's supervision for one or two years, with early fitting of appropriate spectacles. The orthoptist should be available in the place where the 'ophthalmic clinic' is held, whether in a school or a hospital setting and referral of babies from a child health clinic should be encouraged. This is especially important when there is a positive family history of squint.

Educational retardation which results from diminished visual acuity should be reduced by early diagnosis and the successful management of the bespectacled child. The orderly development of visual perception depends on the normal maturation of eye movements and of the ability to fix the gaze, factors to be remembered in the assessment of children with specific reading disabilities. As to the causes of blindness responsible for more than 5 per cent in each age group, an analysis conducted by the Royal National Institute for the Blind in 1962 showed in the 0–4-year-olds 60 per cent due to congenital defects, 10 per cent due to optic atrophy, while at that time retrolental fibroplasia, now a much rarer condition, accounted for 15 per cent. In the 5–14-year age group, 48 per cent resulted from congenital defect and 22 per cent from optic atrophy. Many syndromes and metabolic disorders, all absolutely rare, are associated with varieties of cataract and with pigmentary degeneration of the retina. The effects of some of the inborn errors of metabolism, for example galactosaemia, are preventable. Accident prevention plays its part in reducing burns and local trauma to the eyes.

Spectacles

Between 5 and 6 per cent of the total school population (NCB, Digest of Health Statistics) are prescribed glasses which require revision and servicing (67 000 out of 391 000, some 6 per cent of spectacles provided, needed reglazing in 1969). Davie *et al.* (1972) point out that while 85 per cent of children fitted with spectacles have optimal vision in their better eye, even after correction a substantial number will have sub-optimal vision and will need special supervision in class-room teaching. There is, besides, the unwillingness of some children to tolerate the wearing of spectacles.

DEFECTS OF HEARING AND DISORDERS OF COMMUNICATION, LANGUAGE AND SPEECH

These subjects being closely connected are discussed together. With the decline in acute and chronic infections of the middle ear, the children's 'hearing' clinic has in recent years enlarged its interests to include investigation and treatment both of those children with speech and language disorders which result from defects of hearing and those where there is no gross hearing loss and perhaps not even a defect of auditory perception such as poor auditory discrimination.

The special educational needs of *deaf* children were among the earliest to be recognized and the long tradition of special teaching dates from the Education Act of 1893. The need is determined not only by the degree of hearing loss but also by the quality of the pre-school training, intelligence and cultural background. The segregation of deaf children in special schools and more importantly in residential ones has become less necessary with improvements in living conditions and the increased availability of hearing aids and of special teachers and methods in ordinary day schools. A childhood spent in a residential deaf school may make later integration within a hearing society very difficult. Special teaching for the hearing defect must also be provided for those deaf and partially hearing children whose other handicaps dictate their placement, for example, in training centres for the severely mentally subnormal.

Babies with serious hearing defects need early auditory stimulation if they are to speak normally. Routine screening tests at 6 months in child health clinics, if all families attended, would reveal doutful as well as certain deafness. The reaction of the baby to sounds depends mainly upon the quality of the end organ, but a baby unused to sounds, especially speech sounds, may respond poorly. More precision in diagnosis of deafness in babies can be gained from electroencephalographic studies with Evoked Response Audiometry (Roberts and Watson 1973). Because of the importance of early diagnosis for the baby's future, greater use should be made of such techniques. The 'Memorandum on Deafness in Early Childhood' (Central Health Services Council, HMSO 1971), stated that one child per thousand is born profoundly deaf and the quantity of moderate and of lesser degrees of hearing deficit is several times as great. Among school entrants inspection revealed definite hearing defects in 7.9 per 1000 inspected, while observation was required for 18.3 per 1000, estimated as 6417 and 14 865 in 1971.

Sheridan (1972) reported that in the 1958 cohort of the Perinatal

Mortality Survey assessed at 7 years old, 113 out of 4220 (2.67 per cent) without audiograms showed hearing impediment, while 'significant' decibel loss was noted in 636 of 11 276 presenting full audiograms (5.74 per cent). These were further classified as moderate (35–54 db loss) 4.97 per cent of the total examined, serious (55–74 db loss) 0.48 per cent, and severe (>75 db loss), 0.18 per cent. The loss was unilateral in 474 or 74.5 per cent of those with significant loss. The calculation produced an incidence among 7-year-olds, of those requiring special education, of 2.5 per 1000 of the cohort. Applied to the 7-year-old population in 1971, there should have been no less than 2073 7-year-olds alone in need of special education for defective hearing. Seven-year-old children contribute 10.7 per cent of the total school population (5–14 years). The study also showed that children with severe *unilateral* hearing defects were educationally disadvantaged.

In January 1970 deaf and partially deaf children in special schools numbered 3363 and 1936 respectively. A further 2006 partially deaf children were in special units in ordinary schools, and 232 were receiving part-time education. The prevalence of children needing special teaching was 8 to 9 per 10 000 (n = 8 597 451). The number of pupils in the 49 special schools for the deaf and the partially hearing was 5082. Special educational provision was made for 7979 pupils, including those with multiple handicaps. A service exists for fitting, supervising, servicing and replacing hearing aids. Comparing the NCB cohort prevalence with the actual provision suggests that there was a considerable short-fall in the numbers of children whose hearing deficit had been identified. Possibly some of the hearing deficit was temporary, although this seems unlikely in the severe deficit group.

Two changes are apparent in the last few years. The first is the recognition of 'glue ears', a form of conductive deafness due to secretions in the middle ear. The condition, which is temporary, causes an effective although moderate hearing loss (20 to 40 db) in between 10 and 20 per cent of school children, the rate being highest in heavy industrial towns and lowest in the country (Fuller 1973). Treatment usually begins with removal of the adenoids. Recurrence leads to myringotomy with or without insertion of a ventilating tube. The operation can be done with 24 hours in hospital or with day care only but the ventilating tube needs a monthly inspection until spontaneously extruded in 2 to 12 months. Should 'glue ears' cause a hearing loss at 5 or 6 years of age, the child may find sufficient difficulty in hearing the teacher at school to disturb seriously the programme of learning to read, write and spell.

The same effect may be expected from an auditory perceptual defect now increasingly recognized (and this is the second recent change) in children with normal pure tone audiograms. Defective auditory discrimination is one of the factors contributing to educational problems. Recognition is important so that the child's difficulty is appreciated and so that the child may sit near the teacher who is encouraged to enunciate words with maximum clarity. The prevalence is unknown but, in a small group of boys over the age of 8 years with normal audiograms, poverty of discrimination was demonstrated in between 1 in 5 and 1 in 7 (Naidoo, 1972).

Disorders of speech, language and communication

The ability to communicate is given a lower priority in England and Wales than success in locomotion. This appears a reasonable conclusion to draw from a comparison between the two groups of the amount of attention and assistance given. Much study has gone into the diagnosis of orthopaedic defects, congenital dislocation of the hip, the various types of talipes, spinal deformities, as well as the neuro-muscular disorders and the results of accidents. Special shoes, wheel-chairs, tripods, crutches, besides an army of physiotherapists are available in the National Health Service to assist locomotion.

By contrast, little training is given to doctors about disorders of speech, language and communication except in a few enlightened medical schools. It is taken for granted that the parents will provide the language stimulation needed for the normal development of speech, and delay is tolerated in a way that would not be acceptable in the matter of walking. Yet treatable adverse factors such as inadequate stimulation, most marked when the child is deaf and unable to accept the stimulation, or 'baby-minded' in relative silence, and deprivation, when the child is not living in a family, greatly retard the development of speech (Pringle 1965). In the deprived child, what is 'least affected is neuro-muscular development, including walking, other locomotive activities and manual dexterity. The most affected is speech, the ability to express being more retarded than the ability to understand' (Bowlby 1951). The influence on learning ability is generally agreed to be considerable. Sheridan (1973) reported on 215 children (144 boys and 71 girls) with normal hearing and marked speech defects. Many were later members of large families in lower-income groups, a high proportion born prematurely. Motor and educational achievement were delayed and more than half were attending special schools or receiving remedial teaching. Sheridan makes a plea for improved assessment. The group with marked speech defects was of the same size as that of the children with significant hearing loss.

Much more attention should be paid to this subject in both undergraduate and post-graduate training of doctors as well as in the training of paramedical personnel including nursery nurses. Special clinics for the diagnosis of communication, language and speech problems, the modern form of children's hearing clinic, are essential. Their task is not only the assessment of the child's hearing and general intelligence and the identification of motor or other sensory deficits but also of the family circumstances. The provision of hearing aids and availability of teachers of the deaf will be sufficient for some children. Others will need skilled social support, for language is a social skill. For others remedial education will be required.

Some need the help of speech therapists. In 1971 speech therapy was being provided for 94 000 children in England and Wales, 457 in special schools with 80 more places due. (House of Lords Debate, Hansard, 20 December 1972, 337, 25.) The Quirk Report (1972) recorded that 2 per cent of children require speech therapy at some time and that it would benefit 3 per cent of pre-school children aged $2\frac{1}{2}$ to 5 years. Neligan and Harris (1965) estimate that, on school entry at 5 years, 4500 children have speech and language disorders and although some recover without help, all require expert management. Guidance from experts is needed by parents and teachers.

Mac Keith and Rutter (1972) studying reports from Newcastle, Bristol, Edinburgh and the Isle of Wight conclude 'that 1 per cent of children come to school with a marked language handicap and a further 4 to 5 per cent may show the sequelae of earlier language difficulties'. Applied to 1971 populations the numbers would have been respectively 8000 and from 30 000 to 40 000.

Cerebral palsy and mental handicap are the commonest physical conditions associated with language delay. In autistic children and in those with severe behaviour disturbances, one of the main problems may be difficulty in communication. Language development suffers. The possibility of an underlying hearing deficit has always to be remembered even in a child who is an obvious mongol. The apportionment of blame, when there are communication difficulties, between intellectual impairment, behaviour and personality disorder and deafness may require prolonged observation and repeated testing even in the most experienced hands.

Problems of articulation cause parents sufficient anxiety to lead to visits to doctors. With regard to stuttering most surveys agree that something of the order of 5 per cent of all children are affected at some time under the age of 13 years and that 1 per cent become persistent stutterers. An estimate for 1971 would indicate that some 40 000 school entrants stuttered or were likely to stutter at some time, that 8000 would be added to the numbers of persistent stutterers in the community and that this kind of addition would be likely each year. Andrews and Harris (1964) have summarized current knowledge. If it is agreed that it is probably 'a complex learned habit' which follows some genetic contribution, which begins most often before the age of 5 years, and which, if persistent, evolves into a serious personal problem for the sufferer, more research and informed teaching are essential. The advice of doctors is sought. The present paediatric curriculum does not prepare them to give it.

Immigrant children from non-English speaking countries not only need instruction in the language but some also need speech therapy. This is naturally a larger problem in some areas than in others. The special problems of certain racial groups are noted in Chapter 21.

CHAPTER 7

Dental care

Dental care must be included among the health needs of children, both in practice and in paediatric education. The subject is too important to ignore, although the ways in which the service is provided are matters for the dental profession. 'Dental disease (dental caries and chronic marginal gingivitis) shares with respiratory disease the distinction of being the most common disease in children' (Court and Jackson 1972).

It is estimated that the average 5-year-old starts school with 4 decayed milk teeth. By the age of 15 years on an average 10 out of 28 permanent teeth are decayed, missing or filled. The NHS provides 7000 dentures to school children each year (Royal College of Physicians 1976).

About 250 000 new children need orthodontic treatment each year and this is provided by three NHS dental services, general (78 per cent), school (12 per cent) and hospital and specialist (10 per cent). The treatment seldom starts before 7 years and the majority begin between 9 and 13 years with a mean duration from 13 to 20 months. The demand varies and is greater in the south of England. That the relationship between malocclusion and health is not yet fully determined leaves unclear the part to be played by the doctor supervising the health of children.

On the service side a 'sort of minimum frequency of visits to the dentist' is estimated at six on an average, but regular attenders are expected three times a year. However, even to enable all 3- to 4-year-olds to be seen once a year would need three times the present provision of treatment.

IS DENTAL CARIES PREVENTABLE?

In the recent report, *Fluoride, teeth and health,* a special committee of the Royal College of Physicians of London has reviewed the arguments and the research and has come down unequivocally on the side of the fluoridation of drinking water. The committee accepts the claim that the simple measure of bringing the fluoride level in drinking water during the years of tooth formation up to 1 mg per litre (a level enjoyed now by only half a million of the population) would substantially reduce dental caries through life. Decayed teeth are accepted as an inevitable part of life by parents with the same resignation as were acute specific fevers before immunization and as are still accidents of all kinds. The time seems ripe for all, including parents, who seek to promote child health, to press for this important measure of prevention.

SUGGESTED DENTAL SYLLABUS

Professor G. L. Slack

Discussions with Professors G. L. Slack and D. S. Berman have led to the following recommendations of a suitable syllabus of instruction. An *overall* view should be presented under the following headings:

1 The aims and objectives of dentistry for the child patient.
2 The growth and development of the oral and dental tissues and factors that may affect normal development.
3 Common diseases that affect the oral and dental tissues of children and an indication of their diagnosis and treatment.
4 The dental services available for children.

A more detailed consideration should be given of:

1 The scope of children's dentistry and orthodontics.
2 The stages of normal development of the oral and dental tissues, including:
   - (a) The structure of the tissues
   - (b) Tooth eruption
   - (c) Development of occlusion
   - (d) Anomalies in the size, number and shape of teeth.
3 Common dental diseases:
   - (a) Dental caries.
     Epidemiology—aetiology—histopathology—treatment.
     Sequelae and recognition, with special reference to prevention including fluoridation.
   - (b) Acute and chronic dental alveolar abscess. Diagnosis and treatment. Sequelae.
   - (c) Acute and chronic inflammation of the gingival and oral mucosa.
     Diagnosis and treatment, including acute ulcerative gingivitis, chronic marginal gingivitis, acute herpetic gingivo-stomatitis, aphthous ulceration.
   - (d) Developmental abnormalities:
     - (i) Malocclusion, recognition of marked variation of the normal.
     - (ii) Cleft palate—early stages and treatment.

4 General diseases in relation to dental health:
   (a) Physically and mentally handicapped patients
   (b) Emotionally disturbed children
   (c) Congenital heart disease
   (d) Haemophilia and other bleeding diseases
   (e) Rheumatic heart disease
   (f) Epilepsy
   (g) Effect of drugs on teeth, e.g. tetracyclines.

5 Dental services for children:
   (a) School dental service
   (b) General dental service
   (c) Hospital consultant
   (d) Orthodontist/paedodontist
   (e) Auxiliary personnel
   (f) When, how, to whom to refer.

6 Other topics:
   (a) The role of preventive dentistry
   (b) The use of local and general anaesthesia
   (c) Fear in relation to dentistry.

CHAPTER 8

School health

The details of the actual health needs of school children are easy enough to identify and, because this is a captive population that has been observed for many years, comparatively easy to quantify. Four recent reports, ammunition for the struggle about whose pairs of hands should provide the service, have been studied. These come from the BPA itself (Paediatrics in the Seventies pp. 25–28), from Dr F. Bamford of the Manchester University Department of Child Health, from the late Dr J. D. Kershaw on behalf of the School Health Service Group of the Society of Medical Officers of Health, and, especially valuable because of his 'quantification', from Dr Kingsley Whitmore of the DES. The siren song of integration failed to silence all other voices but the uncommitted observer noted with interest the intensity of the triangular fight between the local authority doctors whose task risked extinction, the general practitioners and the newly involved community based paediatricians, for an activity which had previously neither enjoyed high status nor been regarded as especially attractive. Indeed, when the purposes of the service are re-examined through modern eyes, much of what is needed might be seen to be the job of other professionals than physicians, but if of physicians, then while their preventive work continues, their outlook will need reorientation in the direction of the paediatrics of development, of education and of life and habit. The task is a major one for total child health. Its size is such that no-one with experience can be spared, from whatever category he comes. Analysis of objectives and a logical assignment of the many different elements in the composite whole must lead to administrative changes and basic alterations in training to fit the new pattern of work to be done.

The aim of the school health service at its inception in 1907 was to ensure that school children would not be prevented from securing the benefits of education by reason of ill-health or defect. It was hoped, too, that the detection of existing disease in its early stages would lead to more effective treatment. And, as the years passed, an increasing list of special defects was compiled for which special educational provision was recommended in either special classes or special schools.

At the same time certain children were, unfortunately, classified as ineducable and excluded altogether from the school system. The factors accepted as impeding education became somewhat stereotyped.

In the early days of the service a classical clinical examination, conducted at school entry and often without a history from the parents, allowed only poor hygiene and gross physical disease or defect to be discovered. Re-examination at certain specified ages and a system of follow-up inspections, mainly to learn whether recommended steps had been successful or had actually been taken, fulfilled the doctors' obligations. The following modern list of the school child's health needs shows the extent of the changes that have followed improvement in general health, growth and nutrition, the development of prophylactic immunization, the provision of National Health Service care, which offers free to all the opportunity for medical examination in infancy, and the widening of health horizons.

1 From birth or during the first two years, the paediatrician, the GP and/or the child health centre will have identified much of the defect and disease, mainly congenital but some acquired, that may interfere with normal education.
2 Pre-school developmental assessment examinations will have identified some of the children needing special education by reason of motor, sensory or perceptual handicaps. Particular attention must be paid to defective development of language, speech and communication. The record of pre-school examinations should be available to the school doctor and will become more useful as screening tests increase their predictive accuracy.
3 All school entrants require examination and assessment, either just before or just after entry. This is not now intended as a case-finding exercise so much as an 'occupational' test of fitness for the process of normal education and a pointer to any modification of teaching method needed by the child. The physical state of the pupil, and particularly the neurological competence, remain important, but also included are predictive educational, socio-economic and emotional assessments, since home conditons, deprivations and attitudes towards education are as relevant as defects of sight and hearing.
4 Five streams of pupils will flow from these assessments:
   (a) those judged to be totally normal,
   (b) those with disability or educational difficulty who need some form of remedial help,
   (c) those in need of psycho-paediatric help,
   (d) those in need of medical treatment, much of which should already be in hand,

(e) those whose homes and families provide inadequate support for pupils trying to make good adjustments to education in school.

Among this last group should be included vulnerable children from broken homes, from single parent homes or with mentally handicapped or delinquent parents, deprived children of all types, immigrant children who have not become culturally or linguistically integrated among their fellow pupils. There is no certainty that one child will belong to one stream only.

5 All children need a periodic review of vision and hearing. Visual acuity should be tested annually or in alternate years. Audiometric testing has been recommended at 7, 10 and 13 years. At entry and at 7, 10 and 13 years, height and weight should be measured and feet, back and skin condition surveyed. Hygiene and general cleanliness need continual observation. A screening test for colour vision is advised.

6 As age advances, failure to make expected educational progress should lead to review. This applies both to those previously regarded as totally normal and those in the other streams, as well as to those with a record of frequent absence. The assessment should include both function and aetiology. Mild mental handicap and new home and family situations may then become apparent, and, especially during the seventh and eighth years, specific learning difficulties.

7 Over regular school examination of healthy normal pupils making their expected progress through school, practice varies between education authorities. Dr Kingsley Whitmore, after full consideration of the reported efficiency of routine examinations of whole age groups and examination of children selected by parent, teacher or school nurse, considered that the school entrants examination should be followed by subsequent medical examination only on request. The effectiveness of such a system can be greatly increased by the use of parent and teacher questionnaire, say as children approach 8 and 11 years. There is some discussion whether school leavers should be medically examined or interviewed, but there should always be an opportunity for discussion of health or career problems between the pupil and the doctor, the teacher and the Youth Employment Service.

8 Booster immunization should be given during the school years. Whether this should be done in school or by the GP remains controversial.

9 The head teacher and perhaps his staff should have the opportunity for discussion with a doctor at least once each term on general health topics, health education programmes and on school hygiene, including

prevention of accidents and investigation of outbreaks of infectious disease.

10 Some teaching should be provided on physical and mental health and on hygiene. Were the school doctor involved in teaching such subjects as biology and human relationships, he could be better accepted as a member of the school staff. In this way, the status and the satisfaction of his job would increase.

11 Someone, necessarily a doctor, must supervise liaison with hospitals, family doctors, child guidance clinics over some of the pupils, and time and opportunity for correspondence is essential.

12 All pupils known to be handicapped should be examined not less than once a year.

13 Such pupils, whether in special schools or not, need support in dealing with their handicaps, and their teachers and their parents need discussions, advice and support.

14 The headmaster (with the staff?) of a special school needs to have discussions with a doctor at least twice each term. What needs explaining is the meaning of medical terms, the effect of the handicap on the child's learning and activities, and what progress should be expected. The teaching staff have no right of access to medical reports and should be greatly assisted in their work by these verbal explanations.

15 Special regard must be paid to the interview with the handicapped school-leaver about his future employment.

16 The school population provides opportunities for studying the natural history of diseases and defects and for research. Two obvious areas are orthopaedics and psychiatry. Much attention is now paid to the feet and back, where the limits of normality remain ill-defined. The problems of tobacco, alcohol and other drugs, delinquency and the control of sexual behaviour face adolescents, and presumably the individual's ability to solve these problems reflects attitudes that have formed during school days. The doctor with the health visitor and social worker may be able to arrange periodic group meetings where tobacco, alcohol and drug addiction can be discussed in an informal atmosphere. Sex education, contraception and termination of pregnancy should take their place in the context of homemaking and the responsibilities of life as a member of a family.

17 The minor ailment clinic, run traditionally by the school nurse, is probably unnecessary. What is wanted is a nurse rather than a clinic. The question remains open whether special therapeutic clinics for enuresis or otorhinolaryngology should be conducted on school

premises. The great demand for expert ophthalmological services for school children, may be held to justify continuing this special clinic at least, although the answer must vary from place to place with size of population and availability of alternative centres in hospital or elsewhere.

18 Whoever has the carrying out of these tasks, the medical personnel cannot function efficiently without the help of professional, non-medical colleagues. Of these the relative importance cannot be judged; all are essential—educational welfare officer, health visitor, medical and psychiatric social worker and, not least, educational psychologist. The service also employs a number of special therapists, speech-therapists, physiotherapists, orthoptists and audiometricians.

Tables 8.1, 8.2, 8.3 and 8.4 concern the health needs and the services for school children provided through the schools. Tables 8.1, 8.2 and 8.3 were provided by Dr. Kingsley Whitmore.

Table 8.1. Recorded incidence of certain defects and diseases in 1969 requiring treatment and/or observation

Number of periodic inspections in 1969 – 1 033 846
Number of special inspections in 1969 – 365 640

Defect	Number of defects				
	Entrants	*Intermediate*	*Leavers*	*Special Inspection*	*Total England and Wales*
Skin	27 246	21 895	17 079	51 823	118 043
Eyes — vision	75 771	89 034	65 433	58 730	288 968
squint	21 866	10 237	3 768	6 573	42 444
other	4 606	4 076	2 586	5 571	16 839
Ear — hearing	37 127	18 174	5 121	24 432	84 854
otitis media	19 187	6 851	2 725	3 849	32 612
other	7 419	3 631	1 823	6 757	19 730
Nose and throat	75 399	28 097	9 774	18 007	131 277
Speech	27 547	8 323	1 556	9 094	46 520
Lymphatic glands	19 462	5 426	1 215	3 485	29 588
Heart	14 723	7 488	4 071	4 470	30 752
Lungs	24 289	13 325	5 494	8 060	51 168
Development — hernia	5 629	2 125	581	1 022	9 357
other	22 233	14 143	4 549	8 223	49 148
Orthopaedic — posture	4 758	5 731	4 308	1 910	16 707
feet	28 235	16 903	8 503	9 031	62 672
other	16 427	10 333	6 429	8 257	41 446
Nervous system — epilepsy	3 097	2 783	1 294	1 992	9 166
other	7 700	5 233	1 993	4 562	19 488
Psychological — development	13 535	13 889	3 488	67 518	98 430
stability	26 214	18 687	4 866	13 815	63 582
Abdomen	7 150	5 276	2 195	2 447	17 168
Other	20 992	20 134	9 290	46 009	96 425

Table 8.2. Numbers of school children known to have received certain forms of treatment in England and Wales during the year ending 31 December 1972

	Number of clinics	*Sessions*	*Pupils treated*
Child guidance	498	20 839	74 696
Speech therapy	1 572		103 909
	Uncleanliness and verminous	*Infested*	
Total examinations in schools by authorized persons	12 895 024	266 602	

Table 8.3 Number of certain defects known to have received treatment by the authority or otherwise, however they were brought to local education authorities' notice, whether by periodic inspection, special inspection or otherwise, during 1969

	Number of defects treated, or under treatment during the year 1969		
	England	*Wales*	*Total*
Diseases of the skin:			
Ringworm – scalp	429	3	432
Ringworm – body	722	47	769
Scabies	17 282	1 260	18 542
Impetigo	9 468	239	9 707
Other skin diseases	147 101	3 630	150 731
Eye diseases: Defective vision and squint:			
External and other (excluding errors of refraction and squint)	28 974	628	29 602
Errors of refraction and squint	378 935	25 370	404 305
Number of pupils for whom spectacles were prescribed	191 310	11 058	202 368
Defects of ear:			
Total number of pupils still on registers of schools at 31 December 1969 known to have been provided with hearing aids:—			
(a) during the calendar year 1969	1 858	139	1 997
(b) in previous years	11 657	614	12 271
Convalescent treatment:			
Number of pupils who received convalescent treatment under School Health Service arrangements	6 295	396	6 691
Minor ailments:			
Number of pupils with minor ailments	308 643	4 407	313 050

Table 8.4. Handicapped children receiving education in special schools, independent schools, special classes and units, boarded in homes at January, 1970
(Taken from Annual Abstract of Greater London Statistics)

B = Boarding
D = Day

		GLC	
		Greater London	*Total*
Blind	D	15	
	B	153	168
Partially sighted	D	425	
	B	31	456
Deaf	D	489	
	B	180	669
Partially hearing	D	673	
	B	88	761
Physically handicapped	D	1 595	
	B	303	1 898
Delicate	D	1 703	
	B	514	2 217
Maladjusted	D	1 772	
	B	1 785	3 557
ESN	D	8 353	
	B	1 147	9 500
Epileptic	D	25	
	B	85	110
Speech defective	D	24	
	B	13	37
Total	D	15 074	
	B	4 299	19 373
Total school population			1 089 166

CHAPTER 9

Chronic handicap and long stay residential care

At 30 January 1970 in England and Wales 71 442 children (see Table 9.1) between the ages of 5 and 15 years were being provided with special education because of handicap. The largest single group consisted of

Table 9.1 Education provision for handicapped children aged 5–14 at 30 January 1970, England and Wales
(From Statistics of Education, DES, 1970. Table 29)

Newly assessed	*Newly placed*	*Under 5 years*	*All Pupils*	*%*	*Special Schools 5–14*
135	129	60	1 278	0.016	780
341	303	45	2 292	0.029	1 668
355	379	75	3 576	0.046	2 663
525	515	58	4 403	0.057	1 584
1 903	1 839	284	11 701	0.152	7 007
2 555	2 398	21	9 046	0.111	5 957
3 440	2 681	14	13 360	0.176	5 348
12 271	12 100	72	65 179	0.085	44 857
218	195	1	861	—	815
101	82	3	334	—	763
21 844	20 621	633	112 030	1.46%	71 442
During 1969 children reported unsuitable for education			1 336	Pupils in hospital schools 3 505	
				Under 5	608
Full-time pupils				Aged 5–14	2 645
E & W 5–14 DES			7 668 836	15–19	252

the educationally subnormal (62.7 per cent). Of the remaining 26 585, almost half were classified as physically handicapped (7007) or delicate (5957). The others, those with defective vision and hearing, with seizures and with speech defects and the large group of maladjusted (5348) are discussed under their appropriate headings. No separation is made in the table for cerebral palsied children, who may appear in any of the groups and who are discussed in Chapter 14.

The remainder is made up of a heterogeneous collection of medical and surgical conditions with no doubt a contributing socio-economic component when family life at home is not available or is such that a normal school life is too difficult for the child.

Certain general principles are common to the health needs of children with physical handicaps which either limit mobility or make regular attendance at a day school impossible. It is proposed, following some general remarks, to instance the child with spina bifida as an example of serious chronic handicap associated with multiple defect.

The ultimate aim, which must always be kept in mind when decisions are taken, is to help the child to achieve as much independent living as possible. This will necessitate a collaboration between him, his parents and their advisers and some adaptation of his environment, which includes not only house, furniture and fittings, and facilities for personal hygiene, but also clothes, utensils, books and toys and movement about the house. Doctors play a leading part in all this, especially in the early years and plenty of evidence exists that they do not sufficiently help their patients with obtaining these aids. Timing of help to meet the child's needs to develop is of the utmost importance. The remark, sometimes made when drugs and operations are not appropriate, that there is no treatment is always harmful and never true. Since the defect in the doctor's practice is part faulty attitude and part ignorance, the principles and some of the techniques of the habilitation of babies and children should hold an important place in clinical instruction.

The immediate aim is to ensure that the parents accept the situation as it is and are prepared to co-operate with those helping them. Feelings of guilt, isolation and anxieties about the future need discussion. Many need much detailed instruction in the manipulation of the handicapped child. All need the greatest kindness and consideration over visits to doctors and hospital; their convenience as to timing appointments, their methods of travel, any financial hardship from fares, loss of wages or the payment of minders for siblings should be recognized and understood. Prostheses, chairs, indeed any apparatus should be readily available with an efficient means of servicing and repair in which many fathers would be pleased, with instruction, to play a part. During the school years, surgical operations or periods in hospital should be arranged in relation to the educational programme. If the child needs long-stay management in a hospital school, he must be made ready for life in the world outside (see p. 83 *et seq*. for discussion). Throughout, the child himself needs the love, the acceptance, the security and the confidence which satisfactory emotional development demands. His image of himself must suffer the least possible distortion.

The community has its contribution to make. Roskies (1972) in a study of the mothering of thalidomide children has shown that the mother–child relationship is not the whole. There is in reality a tripartite relationship between mother, child and state. It is the state of which the family is inevitably a part which decides what is normal. Life, in every single aspect, is suited to the 'normal' person. Because handicapped children are born unable to conform to the normal expectations of society, she feels that the state has a special responsibility towards them. This should not be fitful and variable, but should be planned and reliable.

The Attendance Allowance and the possibility of a disablement income are from this point of view completely justified. Nevertheless, it is not only money that counts. The friendliness and understanding of neighbours, help from teachers and later from employers and provision of facilities for the maximum attainment of independent living do as much for human well-being.

SPINA BIFIDA

Under this shorthand title are gathered all the children with multiple congenital defects including meningocele, myelocele, encephalocele and hydrocephalus. There are defects of vertebral development, of the hips and the lower limbs. The spinal cord defect results in a paraplegia with loss of sensation and of control of micturition and defaecation. The urogenital tract may be congenitally abnormal or be damaged because of the neurologically defective bladder, ureteric reflux, posterior urethral obstruction and chronic or recurrent infection. Some babies have congenital heart disease or serious congenital defects in other systems.

Incidence and prevalence

During 1969, 1556 affected infants were born in England and Wales, giving a birth *incidence* of 1.9 per 1000 total births. Geographical, seasonal and social class variations exist. In South Wales an incidence of 4.1 per 1000 total births has been reported, while in London at Queen Charlotte's Maternity Hospital the incidence over 16 years has remained remarkably constant at 1.4 per 1000 births. Conception during the winter months and babies of the lowest social class contribute the higher figures. About one quarter occur among stillbirths and a further 15 per cent die within the first week, the majority within the first few hours. It has been stated that before the modern period of early thorough and total treatment fewer than 16 per cent of live born babies survived to 5 years (Laurence 1966). The most optimistic figures at present show a survival to 5 years of approximately 50 per cent. In the earlier period, as indeed today, much depended on the effectiveness in maternity departments of the general management of newborn babies and especially of their feeding and of the control of nursery infection.

This is well illustrated by the results at Queen Charlotte's Maternity Hospital where survival to the age of 5 years or longer occurs more often, but only from the high figure of 42.8 per cent to 54.5 per cent of affected live born babies when the periods 1950–59 and 1960–65 are compared (Table 9.2). Standards of nursery care were excellent during

Table 9.2. Queen Charlotte's Maternity Hospital. Incidence of myelocele, meningocele, encephalocele
An incidence of 1.1 live births per 1000 total births in both periods

	Total births	*Still-born*	*Live-born*	*Alive in 1970*	*Survival rate percentages of Total births*	*Survival rate percentages of Live births*
1950–59						
Total	30 293	684	29 609			
Affected	43	8	35	15	34.8	42.8
1960–65						
Total	18 610	325	18 285			
Affected	28	6	22	12	42.8	54.5

Survival rates at one year for live born babies with spina bifida with and without hydrocephalus in England and Wales
(CMO's Annual Report, DHSS 1973 for comparison)

	Estimated live-born	*Number dead*	*Percentage of live-born alive at one year*
1954	1 313	1 101	16.1
1960	1 525	1 105	23.7
1966	1 747	694	60.3
1972	1 580	654	58.6

Note :
In 1960 a positive attitude towards survival of multiple handicap babies began to be adopted. The high standards of nursing care, especially in the control of infection, at Queen Charlotte's produce higher than average survival rates for all babies. The improved survival rate after 1960 attributable to special treatment has by comparison been much less.

both periods, but modern preventive treatment of spina bifida began only in the second. The quality of nursery care seems from these figures to be of considerable importance in any discussion of survival rates.

The *prevalence* in school children can be calculated on the assumption that only about one half of the live born babies with spina bifida will reach the age of 5 years. In 1969, 365 (23 per cent) of the total of 1556 were stillborn leaving 1190 survivors. The expectation is that 585 will reach school age. Assuming that this was an average year there should at any one time be somewhat less than 6000 school children with spina bifida aged 5 to 14 years. The extent of physical and mental handicap is difficult to calculate, since a greater or lesser element of selection enters into all reported series. As in so many of the problems of handicapped children long-term studies of whole populations are necessary if accurate estimates of child health needs are desired.

Lorber (1971) has made a praiseworthy attempt to examine the quality of life among survivors as a contribution to the ethical problems of the care of severely multiply handicapped children. Brought face to face with the deformities due to thalidomide, doctors in 1962 felt compelled to examine compassionately their attitude towards children born with other severe physical handicaps. The demands of the parents of children with cerebral palsy during the nineteen-forties had already brought recognition of the needs of that group and of methods of assisting the habilitation of the children. The community's charitable feelings were aroused and help at that time came largely through the organization of voluntary groups and societies.

The challenge in the 1960's was to the National Health Service. Advances in treatment in neurosurgery, orthopaedic surgery and genito-urinary surgery together with improved methods of preventing and curing bacterial infections combined to make possible an improvement in the lot of spina bifida children. Much secondary illness and disability had previously increased their miseries and handicaps and now a great deal had become preventable. Valve insertion could prevent hydrocephalus, muscle slides and tendon transplants could increase the chances of mobility, new medical and surgical resources could preserve renal function through the control of infection and the relief of obstruction in the genito-urinary tract. Above all the emergency removal of the sac and of damaging bony spurs and spikes with 'reconstitution' of the spinal cord seemed capable of preserving a degree of neurological function that would otherwise have been lost during the early hours of life.

The response of the Ministry of Health was to accelerate the establishment of a number of neonatal surgical units for which less urgent pleas had been made for a number of years. The response of many doctors, although not all, was gradually to combine into teams for the full assessment of the needs and for overall treatment of the affected children. For some of these teams the aim was for a limited period of trial so that well based decisions could be reached. Certain doubts existed in the minds of all but the most enthusiastic. How much could really be accomplished that would benefit the child in the long run and what would be the cost? The cost would need to be counted not only in money and Health Service beds and staff, but also in the stress on parents and families of caring for children whose needs for physical and moral support and for repeated hospital attendances and admissions would be great. How much damage would be done to the stability of marriages? Above all, what would be the quality of life and what would life have to offer to the grown-up person with spina bifida?

Once improved treatment had become available and a family's reaction towards this serious problem had changed from unrelieved tragedy to justifiable hope, the momentum to provide the treatment became irresistible. But, although no group has been able to conduct a limited trial, a stage has been reached where a careful review has become essential.

Could the outcome be predicted, selection of patients for full treatment would become possible. Were it certain that the survival of those not given the treatment would be short, the problem would be solved. In theory there is a place for euthanasia as the alternative to total treatment, but such a plan would meet the resistance of most practising doctors. A negative compromise can perhaps be reached by studying the good and bad nursery management techniques associated with differences in survival rates.

Lorber's conclusions from Sheffield (Lorber 1971), which are supported by Colliss's study at Queen Mary's Hospital, Carshalton (Colliss 1972), are that babies can be graded at birth. Lorber has formulated criteria on which, in his view, a just selection of babies for total treatment can confidently be made. These include the degree of paralysis at birth and the level of the spinal defect. Other valuable parameters are the head circumference, the presence of kyphosis and of associated gross congenital anomalies and major birth injuries.

Lorber has studied 1191 affected infants, but for the purposes of grading selected only the 524 who were admitted during the first 24 hours. Survivors aged 2 to 12 years number 41 per cent. The 201 patients in the years 1967 and 1968 have been divided into five grades. Those in the worst grade either had no voluntary muscle activity or hip flexion only. Only 25 out of the 51 have died and all the survivors have hydrocephalus and have averaged five operations each within the first three years. The list of their disabilities makes gloomy reading, only relieved by Lorber's opinion that their life expectancy is short. It would be comforting to believe that complete reliance can be placed on this opinion. He does not believe that the quality of life has been improved sufficiently to merit the distressing and sometimes prolonged hospital treatment carried out. This, too, must remain a matter of opinion.

As regards education, a reasonable prediction for an annual intake of 600 would be as follows: in normal schools 150, in schools for the physically handicapped 390, of whom 130 would be mentally retarded, and in schools for severely mentally and physically handicapped 60. These numbers must be multiplied by 10 for all the affected school children in England and Wales. About half the total would lack bowel control and half would have recurrent urinary infections.

These figures give some idea of the likely need for hospital treatment. Provision has to be made for 600 newborns to be admitted each year within hours of birth for assessment and, if accepted, for excision of the sac and the removal of any bony spurs present. Parents need counselling and contact must be maintained with the mother during the rest of her lying-in period. A proportion of the babies will die at this time either before, during or after operation. Some 85 per cent have the Arnold-Chiari malformation and possibly two thirds of these (340) will need valve insertion. A proportion of these will develop meningitis or ventriculitis, a condition which once established is extremely difficult to eradicate. Some will need revision of the valve. A few, following an acute block, will become blind. Unfortunately, attempts at antibiotic prophylaxis have failed.

Sharrard (1971) states that almost half the babies born with myelomeningocele show no deformity of the lower limbs at birth but many develop secondary deformities involving hips, knees and feet unless active preventive measures are taken. Operations to improve the function of the lower limbs and to make walking with or without aid a useful accomplishment occupy much time in infancy and early childhood. Fractures, especially of the femur, are common in later childhood from seemingly trivial trauma.

Sensory loss combined with paraplegia and urinary incontinence sets the stage for pressure sores. Once these have occurred ulceration tends to be deep and healing may be slow even under optimal conditions. Parents need to ensure that the buttocks and lower limbs are moved and are kept as dry as possible during the twenty-four hours.

The genito-urinary tract may be the site of a congenital anomaly but more commonly there is a secondary dilatation of ureter and renal pelvis associated with posterior urethral obstruction. Retention with overflow and ureteric reflux favour repeated urinary tract infections which occur in as many as 60 per cent. Transurethral bladder neck resection is commonly practised and, later, diversionary operations to transplant the ureters into an ileal loop previously transferred to the abdominal wall. Repeated intravenous pyelograms may be required.

Continued urinary tract infection with outflow tract obstruction may damage the kidneys and lead to uraemia. It is debatable whether renal dialysis and renal transplantation (see pp. 99, 189) should play any part in prolonging life in more than exceptional patients.

Bowel control is less frequently affected. The use of suppositories and of manual removal of faeces have greatly reduced the problem of 'constipation' and faecal incontinence.

Functional loss including visual, auditory and other perceptual systems should be identified by appropriate tests. A complete assessment is essential if the child is to benefit fully from education.

During childhood the morale of the child and of the rest of the family needs much support by social workers and by the exercise of the maximum of consideration by hospital personnel. Out-patient consultations should be well-planned and the welfare of siblings specially regarded during the repeated in-patient periods. Fares and loss of wages may easily cripple family finances. There is besides the physical work of manhandling the paraplegic child whose weight increases with age. A rest for the mother during the child's second year may be critical for the family. While a holiday for the child may not always be desirable, a day centre can be of great value.

Parent counselling is also needed. Aetiology remains obscure. Nevertheless the chance of recurrence exists and increases, from between 5 to 8 per cent for a second, to from 12 to 24 per cent for a third baby. Prediction by studies of alpha-fetoprotein should soon become more accurate and more readily available. Their use when a pregnant woman has already produced an affected baby is essential. Application to the whole population is bound up with the general problem of screening. The development of reliable methods of measurement in blood samples would bring this possibility within range.

For those who survive to adult life the difficulties of achieving independent living, of career and of sex life remain great. Parsons (1972) has studied aptitude assessments at school-leaving age and shown that the young people are slow but accurate in clerical skills and are best in mechanical comprehension, the only untimed test. They are poor at manual precision, due more to delay in execution than in understanding. The most affected are those with hydrocephalus.

Care is needed in the training of nurses and of social workers who work with these children and their families. Those who have experience of very severely handicapped older children will understand better that not every baby should be given every possible treatment. Antibiotics may not always be prescribed for babies with infections who have the severest combinations of handicaps. Decisions should be explained to all members of the treating team. Doctors do not all agree about the extent to which parents should be involved in these decisions.

LONG-STAY HOSPITALS AND BOARDING SCHOOLS

A re-appraisal is long overdue of the purposes of long-stay hospitals and boarding schools and to what extent they fulfil those purposes and adequately meet the health needs of the children who live in them. For a number of children, the only effective home is one of these institutions.

They owe their origin to the circumstances of the late Victorian and early Edwardian era when attention was being focused on the bad socio-economic conditions in which many handicapped children were living and to the limited opportunity for the proper nursing care at home for children with tuberculosis, rheumatic fever and 'debility'. The large hospitals were too heavily committed to the care of children with acute diseases likely to end in either death or recovery to find beds for those with chronic disease or disabling congenital handicaps. When in 1900 Agnes Hunt opened what is now the Robert Jones and Agnes Hunt Orthopaedic Hospital, Oswestry, the idea was not only to give slum children their surgical treatment in country surroundings, but also to give them work and play and preparation for life. Others began as convalescent homes or tuberculosis preventoria or simply as shelters for those for whom no other place was available. That they have performed an invaluable service cannot be doubted, but, with the general improvement in socio-economic conditions and the change in our understanding of what developing children need to prepare them for life, the question must be faced of whether or to what extent they have adapted themselves to the health needs of the children who now occupy them.

For the nature of their population has changed, both as regards the quality of the homes from which they come and the character of the disorders from which they suffer. No longer are these disorders nutritional, such as rickets, coeliac disease, malnutrition, or infective like tuberculosis and rheumatic fever with rheumatic heart disease, or disabilities like bronchiectasis or the effects of anterior poliomyelitis. These are largely prevented or at least controlled and their place is taken by myelomeningocele, Perthes disease, muscular dystrophy, cerebral palsy and asthma. The recognized needs of the mentally handicapped, too, have entirely changed. There remains a number of disabled children for whom life cannot be managed by their own families at home on account of unsuitable socio-economic conditions, inadequate mothering, or intolerable stress on siblings and on family unity. For all of these the priorities are habilitation, education and preparation for living as independently as possible rather than the surgical procedures which should be designed and timed in relation to these ends. The environment must not be merely some place in which to live; it has to be a place where the child can develop and, furthermore, develop to the maximum of his potential.

The DHSS has conducted a survey of those residential schools and homes, which are non-psychiatric, from the results of which some changes in both policy and management appear to be necessary. Only about one third come under any paediatric influence from either a paediatrician or a paediatrically trained general practitioner. If either does pay regular visits, these are more concerned with the diagnosis and treatment of inter-current disease than with general policy. A full assessment of each child on admission to identify all defects including those that make education difficult is not always carried out. Links with social services departments are thin or non-existent. Perhaps most serious of all, the need for the child to keep in touch with his family is not always given its priority, especially when geography and finance make contact difficult. In relation to the general atmosphere, there is the question to what extent a hospital school, that is a hospital with some educational facilities, should now become a boarding school with medical and surgical facilities and with a house mother rather than a ward system of care.

Many institutions admit children with a wide variety of disorders, but there are still special boarding schools for those with defects of sight and those with defects of hearing, for cerebral palsy, epilepsy, orthopaedic conditions, and one school in England and Wales for each of the following – diabetes mellitus, dermatological diseases and rheumatic heart disease. The policy of segregation by defect or disease should be periodically reviewed. In April 1969 a total of 24 494 residential places was available in special schools administered by DES. (Table 9.3.)

The 82 Hospital Special Schools are not included because they were

Table 9.3. Long-stay hospitals and boarding schools
(From list of special schools for handicapped pupils in England and Wales, HMSO, list 42, 1969)

Nature of School	*Number*	*Places for Boys only*	*Girls only*	*Mixed*	*Total places*
Blind	19	203	150	1 080	1 433
Partially sighted	8	100	80	877	1 057
Deaf and partially hearing	22	79	0	2 171	2 250
ESN	135	4 170	1 982	3 574	9 726
Maladjusted	74	2 135	401	527	3 063
Delicate	48	803	401	2 337	3 541
Physically handicapped	50	248	286	2 126	2 660
Diabetes mellitus	1	0	0	50	50
Speech defect	3	0	0	86	86
Epilepsy	6	56	72	500	628
Total	366	7 794	3 372	13 328	24 494

the responsibility of the DHSS. Of these 20 are hospital schools, which are sited in general or general children's hospitals, where long-stay children in the sense in which this term is used should not be living. The numbers of beds is not stated, but some information can be gleaned from the Report on Survey of Long-stay Hospital Accommodation for Children, April 1969, produced by the DHSS already referred to.

The children included were under the age of 15 years and had been or were likely to be in-patients for at least 4 months in non-psychiatric wards. 54 hospitals with 3 or less such patients were excluded, which kept 98 children out of the survey. The 69 hospitals remaining contained at the time 1463 children. Two unfortunate circumstances have spoiled the figures. Firstly, the analysis includes 22 acute general hospitals which answered the questionnaire, while of the 29 orthopaedic hospital schools in the DES list only 15 replied. Some of the missing hospital schools are large and all of them are no doubt well used, so that an estimate of numbers of children cannot really be properly based on this material. But, because trends may be perceived, a short account of the survey results is included. Table 9.4 shows the distribution of the largest groups.

The seven largest units housed 39 per cent of the total. The source of referral was seldom the family doctor (11 per cent) or the local authority (9 per cent). The former used orthopaedic or acute hospitals, the latter the 'other' or less specialized hospital schools. Hospital consultants referred 44 per cent, using especially orthopaedic hospitals, while 34 per cent were transferred from another hospital. At the time of the survey 202

Table 9.4. Long-stay patients
(DHSS Survey in April 1969)

	No.	*Per cent*		*No.*	*Per cent*
Spina bifida	181	12.4	Perthes	180	12.3
Musculo-skeletal	164	11.2	Asthma	119	8.1
Cerebral palsy	117	8.0	'Social'	24	1.6

(14 per cent) of this group of 1463 children were stated not to be in need of hospital medical and nursing care and 124 (8 per cent of the total) could have been living at home were facilities available. The remainder could have been managed in hostel or boarding school accommodation.

Although these figures represent only a proportion of the children in long-stay hospital type of accommodation, the total number, were it known, cannot be large. It is suggested therefore, that, allowing that an urgent placement may at times be necessary, fewer children would need to be deprived of a 'normal' life if plans were more carefully made after full assessment and with co-ordination between medical, social and educational services, and if the hospital attitude and atmosphere gave place to that of an understanding and well run boarding school.

Reports from the social services department are a necessary part of the data on which decisions are taken. A greater amount of attention needs to be paid to preserving the relationship with his parents of the child from whom long-stay in a hospital school is unavoidable. The social services departments can play an important part in preserving these links as well as in securing the adaptation of the family home for occupation by a severely handicapped child.

CHAPTER 10

Hospital paediatrics

Hospital reports including the statistics of both in-patient and out-patient work and classified by hospital department have been prepared in an increasing number of institutions since Florence Nightingale drew attention to their importance in a paper circulated in 1859. A century later, in 1959, the Registrar-General's Office published a Supplement on Hospital In-Patient Statistics in England and Wales for the year 1955 using the ICD of 1948. The data were collected from a form filled for every tenth discharge or death. In recent reports a multiplying factor allows an estimate to be made from the sample for the whole population and diagnoses have been adapted to the new ICD classifications as these have appeared.

The attempt to quantify the number of discharges and deaths of children in hospital has been made through this Hospital In-Patient Enquiry (HIPE). Unfortunately the arrangement of the data according to the three digit ICD categories is far from ideal for the purposes of the present exercise.

The usual problem exists that meaningful figures can only be collected when an eye is kept on precise objectives. The Enquiry had objectives of its own. These were twofold, firstly to assist in the administration of the hospital services by providing information in terms of the diseases treated and the characteristics of the patients who had those diseases, secondly, to provide data which can be of assistance in assessing the amount, distribution and effect of illness in the community. The data quantify certain characteristics of patients and their diseases, but help administration rather than illuminate professional needs. For example the unit is not the patient but the discharge or death; the regions are compared with reference to bed usage and length of stay, and discharges and deaths are analyzed by source of admission.

The quantification of child health needs requires a quite different arrangement of categories if light is to be shed on the work to be done in hospital by different kinds of doctor. To a great extent the doctor's decisions about the use of hospital beds for children will depend upon the objectives that he seeks to attain. These may be described, in terms of purposes for which admission is ordered, as follows:

(1) Emergency or acute illness when the nature of treatment makes it unsafe for any other course or environmental conditions rule out treatment at home. Factors involved include technology of treatment, i.e. surgical operation, intensive care, or the risk that an emergency might arise necessitating such special measures.
(2) Chronic or recurrent illness for diagnosis, assessment or immediate stabilization of therapy likely to be prolonged.
(3) Chronic handicapping conditions for assessment of function and as a prelude possibly to long stay hospital or residential school placement.
(4) Observation when symptoms and signs are of uncertain significance especially when no other course of action seems available.
(5) Irresistible pressure by parents or otherwise unresolvable anxiety in the doctor's mind.

Both the urgency of admission and its duration are directly related to these purposes. The needs of teaching, of controlled observation and of research for the maintenance and the improvement of the standards of medical practice must be faced. A society, unprepared to accept these needs, accepts as the corollary a declining standard of care. On the other hand the paediatrician more than any other doctor always weighs up carefully the necessity for investigation in depth, bearing in mind that routine investigation is to be discouraged unless some specific purpose is intended. There is always discomfort for a child and sometimes risk.

The dangers and disadvantages of admitting children to hospital and thereby of separating them from their homes and families are now well recognized and steps are taken to reduce them by arranging for the mother to accompany her child, for frequent and convenient hospital visiting and for occupation, education and entertainment of the patient. Hospital admission is an incident in the life of a child, albeit both important and stressful. It may assume priority at one or more times during childhood, but, except in the most serious or in fatal diseases, the priority is short-lived. Hospital consultants and nursing staff, trained in hospitals and with their professional lives centred on hospitals, have to make a positive effort to see the child patient in the context of where he belongs, which is at home with his family or at school with his fellows and his teachers. If this effort is difficult for doctors in general, as it undoubtedly is, the necessity for it forms one of the main reasons why the management of children in hospital requires for its fulfilment a special paediatric orientation. And this can best be provided by a paediatrically trained staff working in a special paediatric department.

That this is still not recognized in practice is shown plainly in Table 5 of the DHSS Census of Children in non-psychiatric hospitals conducted on 7 October 1970, when 2921 children were in adult wards, 1760 with segregation and 1161 without. This amounts to one fifth of the children occupying hospital beds on that night, an improvement no doubt over previous figures but still leaving too many children in accommodation other than that specifically organized for the care of children. As is to be expected the majority of these (2057 or 70 per cent) were in surgical, ENT, ophthalmic, and orthopaedic wards where a case can be made for special nursing and management. Such a case is difficult to make for admission to a general medical ward. That as many as 30 per cent of the children in hospital who were not in children's accommodation were in general medical wards is indeed disappointing.

This is not to say that the paediatrician alone can or should deal with all the hospital problems of children. For most of the children admitted to hospital, the tables derived from HIPE show that the technical part of treatment and often the complete diagnosis call for a specialist, be he surgeon or organ or system physician. A rearrangement of the HIPE statistics would be necessary in order to obtain the true picture of these specialized needs. This has not been attempted in full, because the diagnostic data are not sufficiently accurate and the diagnostic divisions lack the necessary refinement. Too many classes contain large numbers under the headings 'other specified' and 'other unspecified'. Nevertheless the tables give some indication of need.

Table 10.1 lists in order of size the ICD classes I to XVII according to the total estimated discharges and deaths in thousands (HIPE for 1971 Table 5). The composition for each of these classes is discussed in some detail below and the numbers illustrate the practical importance of a relatively few conditions. In Table 10.2, the attempt has been made to rearrange the data according to the main aetiological agent, such as infection, bacterial and viral, neoplasm, malignant and benign, and Table 10.3 arranges the data in relation to the kind of specialist or special department needed to provide the main service for the patient. For example among diseases of the genito-urinary system, urinary infections need a general paediatrician, Wilms' tumours a paediatric surgeon, an oncologist, and a radiotherapist, and acute and chronic renal failure a paediatric nephrologist.

These tables by the nature of the data from which they are derived are very far from being accurate, nor are they complete. They are included to direct attention to the importance of giving thought to fresh methods of recording and analyzing hospital data so that estimates can

Table 10.1. Estimated total number of discharges and deaths in thousands from HIPE for 1971 Table 5 (ICD classification 1965) and percentage of total contributed by each class

		No.	*Per cent*
VIII	Diseases of the respiratory system (460–519)	205.6	23.9
XVII	Accidents, poisoning and violence (800–999, Y60–79)	142.7	16.6
VI	Diseases of the nervous system and sense organs (320–389)	83.8	9.8
IX	Diseases of the digestive tract (520–577)	75.7	8.8
XVI	Symptoms and ill-defined conditions (780–796)	68.1	7.9
XIV	Congenital anomalies (740–759)	60.9	7.1
XV	Certain causes of perinatal mortality and morbidity (760–779)	59.7	7.0
I	Infective and parasitic diseases (000–136)	45.3	5.3
X	Diseases of genito-urinary system (580–629)	39.1	4.5
XII	Diseases of the skin and subcutaneous tissues (680–709)	16.3	1.9
III	Endocrine, nutritional and metabolic diseases (240–279)	16.2	1.9
XIII	Diseases of the musculo-skeletal system and connective tissue (710–738)	14.7	1.7
IV	Diseases of blood and blood forming organs (280–289)	11.5	1.3
II	Neoplasms (140–239)	10.7	1.2
V	Mental disorders (290–315)	4.0	0.5
VII	Diseases of circulatory system (390–458)	2.7	0.3
XI	Complications of pregnancy, childbirth and the puerperium (630–678)	1.0	0.01
		858.0	99.71

Table 10.2. ICD Classes rearranged by conventional aetiology
Estimated total deaths and discharges in thousands (HIPE 1971 Table 5)

Infections	209.2
Trauma	140.5
Congenital	135.8
Allergic	14.4
Haematological	13.1
Neoplasm	10.7
Neurological	9.5
Metabolic	9.0
Nutritional	7.7
Psychiatric	3.7
Endocrine	0.9
Sub-total	541.2

Table 10.3. Estimated case loads derived from HIPE Table 5
The case is credited to the doctors mainly responsible for treatment (see p. 89)

Physician	156 121	Oto-rhino-laryngologist	137 956
Neonatologist	52 281	Surgeon	117 406
Chest physician	19 611	Neurosurgeon	52 022
Cardiologist	18 402	Orthopaedic surgeon	49 184
Haematologist	12 682	Ophthalmologist	29 274
Neurologist	8 656	Genito-urinary surgeon	16 092
Dermatologist	5 871	Plastic surgeon	11 052
Nephrologist	1 975	Dental and oral surgeon	6 731
Endocrinologist	755	Thoracic surgeon	1 478
Metabolic specialist	523	Vascular surgeon	140
Obstetrician and gynaecologist	1 835		
A combined team	7 652		

become possible about the likely work load of different specialist consultants. From Table 10.1 it can be seen that respiratory diseases provide 23.9 per cent and accidents, poisoning and violence 16.6 per cent of the total, so that these two classes comprise over 40.5 per cent. Even a brief analysis of the component parts of this grouping reveals some of the fundamental problems met in constructing a useful classification of diseases. Examination of Class VIII (diseases of the respiratory system) shows that almost half (46.8 per cent) of the children are labelled hypertrophy of the tonsils, and presumably the majority of the estimated 96 158 were admitted to hospital under the care of laryngologists for tonsillectomy. A general feature that produces anomalous results is the mixture within the ICD arrangement of system-related diagnoses with aetiological-agent-related diagnoses. The result is the virtual exclusion of upper and lower respiratory tract infections from the infective diseases and of brain tumours, classed as neoplasms, from diseases of the nervous system.

What follows is a series of short discussions of the ICD classes based on the numbers of discharges and deaths recorded in HIPE associated with the deaths from RGSR which include deaths outside hospital also. Many of the conditions are more fully discussed in the chapters to which reference is made.

Class I. Infective and parasitic diseases (ICD 000–136)

HIPE records 45 333 discharges and deaths in this variegated class, which includes those children admitted to hospital with acute specific fevers, alongside those with intestinal parasites, hepatitis and all forms of tuberculosis. Many important infective conditions appear under systems of which the infected organ is a part. Diarrhoeal diseases (21 692) outweigh all others, especially when added to them are salmonella infections (864) (which are not all necessarily diarrhoea patients), bacillary dysentery (1406) and enteritis due to other specified organisms (1473) giving a total of 25 435.

Intestinal infective disease caused 419 deaths, 327 (78 per cent) of them in the first year and a further 46 (11 per cent) in the second year. Diarrhoeal disease (ICD 009) caused 347 of the deaths (82.8 per cent), and a further 58 (13.8 per cent) resulted from 'enteritis due to other specified organisms' (ICD 008). Only 3.4 per cent of diarrhoeal deaths were from diagnosed bacillary dysentery and salmonella infections. It would be of interest to know the circumstances of death, such as the standard of home care and feeding in these dead babies and whether they were treated at home or in hospital. That 163 died within the first two months, 57 of them in the first four weeks, raises the question of the competence of the babies' immunity responses.

The main contribution to acute specific fevers (5548) came from measles (2181), responsible for 27 deaths. The prevalence of measles should diminish following the success of the immunization programme. Infective hepatitis (1207) with 18 deaths and infective mononucleosis (675) brought the number to 32 865 out of the total for the whole group of 45 355. The remaining groups of any size were tuberculosis of all forms (1373 with 11 deaths), meningococcal infection (797 with 102 deaths, over half in the first year of life) and aseptic meningitis (1827 with 5 deaths). The late effects of anterior poliomyelitis (177) which might well need chiefly orthopaedic care are classed next to the acute disease (66). Moniliasis (443), acariasis (520) and pediculosis (22) were presumably not the basic reasons for hospital admission. Venereal disease still features, congenital syphilis (22) with the nature of the clinical illness unspecified, if indeed these were not children with positive blood tests only (can congenital syphilis now rank as a sexually transmitted disease, the current name for venereal disease?), gonococcal infection (22) and other venereal diseases (22).

RGSR records 805 deaths from infective and parasitic diseases of which 563 (69.9 per cent) died before the first birthday. More than half of these early deaths (327 or 58.0 per cent) were caused by diarrhoeal disease, the other important fatal infections being meningococcal infections 59, septicaemia 66, viral encephalitis 19, adding up to 25.6 per cent. Whooping cough caused 22 deaths in the first year, 20 of these in the first 8 weeks. Measles struck later with 27 deaths, only 6 of which occurred before the age of one year. No deaths were recorded from cowpox or smallpox.

Class II. Neoplasms (ICD 140–239)

HIPE records 10 774 deaths and discharges, divided into malignant (4551) and benign (6223). The solid malignant tumours are discussed in some detail in Chapter 17. As far as hospital discharge during the year 1971 is concerned only a few sites are numerically important. The figures represent discharges and *not* the number of separate patients. The main sites are the eye (321 with 5 deaths), brain and nervous system (509 with 210 deaths), and unspecified urinary organs (388) which presumably include Wilms' tumours. Deaths from malignant neoplasms of the kidney numbered 44. Hodgkin's disease with only 11 (estimated) females accounted for 255 (15 deaths), myeloid leukaemia for 266 (75 deaths), and other types of leukaemia for 1882 (257 deaths), lymphosarcoma for 166, with 42 deaths and bone neoplasms for 188 with 27 deaths. The remaining 554 appear under seventeen headings. The registered deaths from malignant neoplasms amount to 762, and there are another 41 of unspecified nature.

The benign neoplasms occurred mainly in the skin (1096), as haemangioma and lymphangioma (1694) and in bone and cartilage (1063). The remaining 2359 appear under twenty headings. RGSR records 34 deaths; 8 occurred from haemangioma within the first two months and 9 from central nervous system tumours.

Class III. Endocrine, nutritional and metabolic diseases (ICD 240–279)

The HIPE total is 16 222. RGSR records 272 deaths.

This is a heterogeneous collection with very different medical requirements which should be discussed separately. Diabetes mellitus, with 4064 discharges including 25 deaths, is traditionally the responsibility of therapeutic experts in the management of this disease rather than general paediatricians or general practitioners. A period of ward observation is considered necessary either as an emergency because coma was the presenting clinical feature or to establish the need for insulin treatment and to adjust diet and dosage in a child who has a less dramatic illness. The follow-up supervision is discussed in Chapter 17. Most children's hospitals have special clinics where are gathered all children requiring dietary supervision as part of treatment. Cystic fibrosis (see Chapter 17) is not specifically mentioned in HIPE but is included in 'other and unspecified congenital disorders of metabolism (ICD 273)' which caused between them 1295 discharges and deaths. RGSR attributes 131 deaths to cystic fibrosis, 71 per cent in the first year of life. 'Disorders of pancreatic internal secretions other than diabetes mellitus' total 830, and some congenital disorders of metabolism, amino-acid (255), carbohydrate (299), and lipid (55), with 'the other and unspecified' group make a total of 2734.

The purely endocrine group includes disorders of thyroid (321) mainly cretinism, polyglandular dysfunction (222), and disorders of parathyroid (11), pituitary (133), adrenal (133), testis (66) and ovaries (22), a total of 908.

The largest single group, 'other nutritional deficiency' (ICD 269) needs to be broken down into some elements. Of the 6832, only 454 are 5 years old or over. That such a vague title is given to some 65.8 per cent of all the children under the age of 5 years in Class III renders the tables useful only for the few named diagnoses, although possibilities of omission through inexact diagnosis exist even in these.

Class IV. Diseases of blood and blood-forming organs (ICD 280–289)

Discharges and deaths in this class total 11 516, the main constituents being (ICD 287) purpura and haemorrhagic conditions (1949), (ICD 282) hereditary haemolytic anaemia (1595 with 13 deaths), (ICD 286) coagulation defects (1251 with 3 deaths), (ICD 284) aplastic anaemia (255 with 15 deaths), (ICD 280) iron deficiency anaemia (440), and (ICD 285) other unspecified anaemia (465). The coagulation defects affected only 99 females. In Class IV also, 32 per cent of the total are classified as (ICD 289) 'other diseases of blood and blood-forming organs' (5315 with 6 deaths). Leukaemia is classified in Class II (ICD 204–7).

Class V. Mental disorders (ICD 290–315)

The classification of mental disorders is notoriously difficult. Pure mental retardation even in its severe forms is unlikely to require admission to a children's hospital or unit in its own right, that is to say unless complicated by physical disorder of another kind. Out of the HIPE class total of 4008 discharges it is not surprising to find only 930 under this heading (ICD 310–315), although here are found all the 14 deaths recorded by RGSR. The commonest heading is 'behaviour disorders' (ICD 308) (1118), more than twice as many in the under than in the 5 years and over group. Physical disorders of presumably psychogenic origin (ICD 305) number 365, only 44 under five years.

This does not appear to be an important group, and unfortunately the non-existence of satisfactory out-patient classifications and records prevents any real assessment of the amount of hospital time or personnel required nowadays in connexion with mental disorders. A more realistic approach will be found in the discussion in Chapter 13.

Class VI. Diseases of the nervous system and sense organs (ICD 320–389)

The main headings in this class have been traditionally linked in text books of physiology and since the Registrar-General's first 'Statistical Nosology' of 1838. In any discussion connected with the organization of medical and surgical treatment the class is an absurdity. Even when conditions affecting the eye, sight and the conjunctivae (ICD 360–379) and those affecting the ear and hearing (ICD 380–389) are separated, the remainder include a few more infections, alongside epilepsy, migraine, sciatica and omitted are all the neoplasms.

In general central nervous system disorders (ICD 320–358), totalling 11 848 with 534 deaths, the chief component is epilepsy, which includes all the infants discharged after admission with seizures. These (ICD 345) number 5547, 2148 under and 3399 of 5 years and over, contributing about one half of the group and 53 deaths, one tenth of the total. There were 184 deaths from meningitis, 45 per cent with no organism specified. 26 deaths are recorded for the encephalitis group. Meningitis (ICD 320) numbers 1927 and encephalitis (ICD 323) 354. Hereditary and familial disorders (ICD 330–333) number 354 with 72 deaths and cerebral palsy (ICD 343–4) 1938 with 57 deaths. About 30 per cent of deaths occurred within the first year of life and possibly survival would have increased the number of children with severe mental retardation.

Among ophthalmic disorders (32 721 with 1 death) strabismus (ICD 373) has 26 808, evenly divided between the sexes and fractionally more common over the age of 5 years. The surgical treatment of children with strabismus provides one of the main examples of procedures requiring the admission of great numbers of young children to hospital. The services of the ophthalmologist were certainly needed for 1716 more children including those being treated for cataract (631) and detachment of retina (266). Some would almost certainly not have needed ophthalmic specialist care, the diagnosis being an inflammatory condition of the conjunctivae, the eyelids and the lacrymal apparatus (2071), presumably treatable by a general paediatrician, assuming that there were reasons why the general practitioner could not treat the child at home. There remains a group of 2126 that might have needed special ophthalmic care being classed (ICD 378) as 'other diseases of the eye'.

Discharges after admission for aural conditions (ICD 380–389) totalled 39 220 with 48 deaths. This is another unbalanced group, infection providing the largest number. Otitis externa (ICD 380) numbers 440, otitis media with and without mastoiditis (ICD 381–384) under 5 years 7408, and 5 years and over 8238, a total of 15 646. Deafness other than (ICD 388) deaf mutism (22) numbers 1473 under 5 and 11 216 5 years and over. All but 4 of the deaths are attributed to otitis media and 3 out of 4 had died in their first year.

Class VII. Diseases of the circulatory system (ICD 390–458)

HIPE estimate for discharges and deaths is 2757, and RGSR records 204 deaths, 72 (35 per cent) in the first year. The subgroups are active rheumatic fever (553) with 3 deaths, chronic rheumatic heart disease (144), hypertensive disease (77) with 3 deaths and other heart disease (731) with 104 deaths. Cerebrovascular disease (609) includes some intracranial haemorrhages and RGSR records 65 deaths. Diseases of arteries, arterioles and capillaries number 110 with 8 deaths, 5 in the first 8 weeks from arterial embolism or thrombosis. Diseases of veins and lymphatics and other diseases of the circulatory sytem are estimated at 542 with 8 deaths.

Rheumatic disease in its acute form including chorea (110) and resulting valvular disease of the heart is seen as unimportant in number both for morbidity and mortality. Most affected children would be admitted to hospital. The General Practice Report (GPR) records only 11 children none of whom was seen at home. The two important sub-groups, 'other heart disease' and cerebrovascular disease, contain chronic disease of endocardium (ICD 424) 177 estimated discharges and deaths and 16 deaths, cardiomyopathy (ICD 425) with 89 and 33 deaths, and symptomatic heart disease (ICD 427) with 465 and 24 deaths. Myocardial insufficiency caused 11 deaths (only 1 case in HIPE sample equals 11 estimated). Subarachnoid haemorrhage (ICD 430) numbered 166 with 18 deaths under 1 year and total deaths of 38, and cerebral haemorrhage (ICD 431) 255 with 11 deaths. In the final group varicose veins accounted for 77 and haemorrhoids for 100. In the list of operations, those on veins numbered 144 and on haemorrhoids 44.

The health needs of children with congenital cardiovascular anomalies are considered in Chapter 16.

Class VIII. Diseases of the respiratory system (ICD 460–519)

This somewhat mixed class numbering 205 592 represents 23.9 per cent of the total discharges and deaths. A lack of balance is caused by the presence of the group 'hypertrophy of tonsils and adenoids' (ICD 500), which contributes an estimated 96 158, or 46.8 per cent of the whole class and 11 per cent of the year's total estimated discharges and deaths. The list of operations (HIPE Table 22i) gives the higher figure of an estimated 120 983 operations on tonsils and adenoids, 15.5 per cent being performed below the age of 5 years. RGSR records 4 deaths.

The sub-headings in the Class are acute respiratory infections (ICD 460–466) 54 590 with 127 deaths, influenza (ICD 470–474) 509 with 22 deaths, pneumonia (ICD 480–486) 11 748 with 1782 deaths, bronchitis, emphysema and asthma (ICD 490–493) 21 592 with 146 deaths, 'other diseases of upper respiratory tract' (ICD 501–508) and excluding ICD 500, tonsil and adenoid hypertrophy), 14 827 with 56 deaths and other diseases of respiratory system (ICD 510–519) 6245 with 55 deaths.

The acute respiratory infections classified are the common cold (1617), acute sinusitis (122), acute tonsillitis (18 370) with 10 deaths, and acute pharyngitis (1805) with 2 deaths. Acute laryngitis and tracheitis (3167) with 44 deaths should include the children with acute laryngo-tracheo-bronchitis. Twenty-five of these deaths occurred in the first six months and 81 per cent of the discharges and deaths were of children under 5 years. Acute bronchitis and bronchiolitis (ICD 466) is estimated at 8316, 93 per cent under age 5 years, RGSR records 778 deaths, which is 25.4 per cent of all childhood deaths from respiratory disease (3060). The first year of life is the most dangerous, 43 deaths are reported in the first month, 574 before 6 months (73.8 per cent) and 691 before 1 year (88.8 per cent of 778 deaths). Influenza (509) is shown as a rare hospital diagnosis; GPR records 310 consultations among 1 in 167 of the total child population. RGSR records 22 deaths.

Pneumonia due to virus (177), pneumococcus (3311), other specified and unspecified bacteria (310) and acute interstitial (22) accounts for few (3820) estimated discharges from and deaths in hospital. RGSR records 169 deaths from viral, 64 from pneumococcal and 37 from other bacterial pneumonia with 38 deaths from acute interstitial pneumonia making 78 per cent of the deaths in babies less than a year old. 73 per cent of estimated hospital discharges and deaths were in the 0- to 5-year-old age group. More than twice as many (7928) are in the groups bronchopneumonia and pneumonia unspecified, and deaths in the two groups amount to 1474. Out of all the pneumonia and broncho-pneumonia deaths, 343 were within the first month. Some of those would certainly have been late results of respiratory problems at birth and some may well have been in babies with cardio-vascular failure, which imitates the clinical picture of lower respiratory tract infection in this age period. Subtracting these from the 1421 pneumonia deaths in the first year of life leaves 1078, 39.7 per cent of the total deaths from respiratory tract infection.

The next sub-group (ICD 490–493) introduces respiratory allergies: asthma 12 335 (57 per cent of the sub-group) with 58 deaths, unqualified bronchitis 8548 with 71 deaths, chronic bronchitis 575, and emphysema 33 with 17 deaths between them.

Figures for peritonsillar abscess are 155, no deaths recorded. The remainder of this group provide work for the oto-rhino-laryngologist: chronic pharyngitis and naso-pharyngitis (4108), chronic sinusitis (3743), deflected nasal septum (543), nasal polyp (387) and chronic laryngitis (33). Hay fever (709) is a somewhat surprising discharge diagnosis (no deaths). The usual group of 'other diseases', this time of the upper respiratory tract, total 5692. There were 16 deaths in the first 8 weeks of life, 51 in the first 5 years and 55 in all.

Chapter 16 contains a more detailed discussion of the problems of respiratory disorders.

Class IX. Diseases of the digestive system (ICD 520–577)

Three main categories supply 62 385 (82.0 per cent) of the total discharges and deaths of 75 684 in this class, diseases of the oral cavity, salivary glands and jaws (14.4 per cent), appendicitis (38.4 per cent) and hernias and intestinal obstruction (30.8 per cent). What appear to be purely dental or maxillo-facial problems, which will not be considered further, amount to 10 010 with 4 deaths. Cleft palate is included under congenital anomalies (Class XIV).

A full discussion of appendicectomy, appendicitis and hernia is given in Chapter 16, where it is convenient to consider together the other headings in this class.

Class X. Diseases of genito-urinary system (ICD 580–629)

This class numbering 39 077 and contributing only 108 RGSR deaths can be divided into four groups. Outweighing all the rest and providing 51.9 per cent of discharges with no deaths is ICD 605, called redundant prepuce and phimosis (20 285). Surprisingly 41.0 per cent of this large number come into the 5–14-year age group. No doubt many babies are not admitted to hospital for circumcision, and ritual circumcisions are often performed at home. If the older children need admission for paraphimosis perhaps an earlier decision not to circumcise was wrong. It would be valuable to examine the indications for late circumcision when para-phimosis is not the reason. Although the mean stay in hospital is no more than 1.8 days for ages 0–4 and 2.5 days for ages 5–14, nevertheless this single condition is responsible for a considerable use of hospital beds.

In the record of operations (HIPE Table 22i) the figure for circumcision is even higher (21 349). And the operation was performed over 4000 times in the age group 15 to 44 years. For young babies, medical circumcision by means of the plastic bell is available. No record exists of how widely this is being used and with what success. Refinement of diagnosis as to what constitutes redundancy and of indications for circumcision would seem desirable. A further 6.7 per cent (2635) result from the treatment of hydrocele, under age 5 years in 60 per cent. Highly skilled surgical personnel would not seem needed for circumcision nor for the treatment of hydrocele, accounting together for 58.6 per cent of this class.

On the other hand surgeons with special experience do seem to be needed for the management of children with hydronephrosis (565), urinary calculi (255), stricture of the urethra (388) and some part of those with other diseases of the kidneys and ureters (753). There were 277 discharges for orchitis and epididymitis. The second largest number is in the group of 'other diseases of male genital organs' (3675) with one death. How many of these were surgical is not known.

The third group, of medical conditions in which there is some place for renal transplants as well as for renal dialysis, includes acute nephritis (221) with 10 deaths, nephrotic syndrome (720) with 15 deaths, and various forms of chronic nephritis (543) with 14 deaths. Infections of the kidney (564) contribute the largest number of deaths (212) in the whole of Class X, of which 11 occurred in the first month.

Diseases of the breast total 330 for males and females. Disorders and diseases of the female genital organs (the fourth group) account for 1273 with one death. This includes 509 in the 5–14 age group for disorders of menstruation.

A further discussion of diseases of the genito-urinary system will be found in Chapter 16.

Class XI. Complications of pregnancy, childbirth and the puerperium (ICD 630–678)

The obstetric problems of girls under the age of 15 years are increasing. They could only diminish if sex problems could be solved by sex education, contraception and the availability of termination of pregnancy. At present, school sexual *mores* frequently include sexual intercourse. And example rather than precept determines the issue. A case for control of sexual drives for children does not seem to be acceptable to parents, teachers or the children themselves, only control of the result.

Schoolgirls often reveal pregnancy late, do not always wish for termination even when there is time, and prefer to keep their babies rather to have them adopted. More precise knowledge of the aetiology of precocious pregnancy, from both the female and male viewpoints, since a father must be involved, might lead to more effective methods of prevention, but whatever is done, obstetric management is likely to be needed for an increasing number of young single girls unless attitudes change.

In HIPE 1969 there were 701 girls under 15 years old in Class XI, of whom induced abortion accounted for 389 and the delivery of a baby for 291. For comparison the HIPE 1971 figures give 974 girls under 15 years in Class XI, with an increase of induced abortions to 720 and a decline in deliveries to 177. The number of pregnant schoolgirls discharged from hospital has increased by nearly one third in the two years and is increasing.

A somewhat more impressive record of the changes which are now occurring may be found in the 'supplements on abortion' published by the Registrar-General. Unfortunately these figures relate to girls under 16 years not 15 years. Between 1969 and 1973 the number of terminations for these girls has trebled (1231 to 3660), as had the number at all ages, and there are beginning to be girls of 16 who have had two previous live born babies. In 1973 two 13-year-olds, three 14-year-olds and twenty-one 15-year-olds had previously had one live or stillborn baby. There is as yet no record of the numbers of previous terminations of pregnancy. That this is information which should be available is suggested by the steady lowering of the age at which first pregnancies are being terminated (Table 10.4).

Table 10.4. Number of girls by age having terminations noting previous live born children
(RGSR Supplement on abortion Table 7A)

Year	1969		1971		1973	
Previous live-born baby	0	1	0	1	0	1
Aged 10	–	–	–	–	1	–
11	2	–	3	–	4	–
12	7	–	16	–	14	–
13	38	–	77	–	106	2
14	275	2	527	2	693	3
15			1 659	8	2 248	21

The pregnancies are now managed in obstetric units where the patients, married and unmarried alike, are liable to be called Mrs, an appellation greatly resented by the young unmarried girls. The quality of life for the girl and her baby depends on the accuracy with which needs are matched by management and treatment at this critical time, so critical for the families involved as well as for mother and baby. Much could be said in favour of the concentration in one area special obstetric unit of experience about these families, their social needs, the problems of adoption, of continuing education for the girls and of future prospects which could form the basis for improvements both in tactics and strategy. Such a unit could with advantage be linked with an Adolescent Unit with care provided for many of the older girls with sexual problems up to the age of 18 years. This would produce a unit of viable size.

With regard to termination of pregnancy, Wynn and Wynn (1972) have gathered together from world sources a body of evidence about the effects of abortion upon subsequent marriage. There is a 2 to 5 per cent risk of sterility, a significant increase in the risk of a stillborn or premature or abnormal child and a loss of efficiency of the cervix. There may be two and a half times the number of premature births for women whose first pregnancy has been terminated. The husband's realization that these difficulties, bad enough in themselves and ones which prevent him from having a normal family, result from the termination of previous illegitimate pregnancy, may stress the marriage to breaking point. And it is the young single girl who is particularly at risk. The only humane decision, short-term, for the pregnant schoolgirl appears to be termination. Long-term follow-up studies are urgently required about the future of both mother and baby. Meanwhile an abortion mortality rate of about 16 per 100 000 (17 per 100 000 maternal mortality rate for England and Wales in 1970) must not be forgotten.

Preventive social work and education can only succeed if it be first accepted that a pregnancy under the age of 15 years is evidence that something other than the contraceptive method has failed. Is sexual intercourse at so early an age to be included in the pattern of normal good health? Is this something desired by the parents or the community for these young girls? No one would dispute that the health needs of children demand that each generation of girls and boys should be capable of producing and rearing normal healthy children. Too early a pregnancy raises problems that are virtually insoluble for both mother and baby. The induced abortion of schoolgirls militates against later success in child rearing. As to prevention, it can only follow a better understanding of what leads children to seek solutions for their life problems through precocious sexual intercourse. The argument between nature and nurture can never be solved. Nevertheless however strong are the impulses that lead children into early sexual experience, and however much genetically determined, their control must be influenced by the emotional experiences of childhood. It is here that all doctors working with families, be they general practitioners or paediatricians whether community or hospital-based, have a part to play.

Class XII. Diseases of the skin and subcutaneous tissues (ICD 680–709)

HIPE records 16 277 discharges and deaths, and deaths number 11, 6 of them under 1 year and apparently due to infection. The infections form 41.3 per cent (6732) and eczematous conditions 19.8 per cent (3222). Almost one tenth (9.8 per cent) are attributed to 'diseases of nail' (ICD 703). There is a surprisingly large number with psoriasis (864) of whom 70 per cent (598) are girls of 5 to 14 years.

Class XIII. Diseases of the musculo-skeletal system and connective tissue (ICD 710–738)

HIPE records 14 727 discharges and deaths, and deaths number 16, in which infection plays an important but unidentifiable part. Osteomyelitis and periostitis, with 2026 discharges and deaths, claimed 3 deaths, although acute pyogenic arthritis with 531 caused no deaths. Chronic arthritis and rheumatoid conditions with 1 death accounted for 1251. Osteochondrosis (2635) gave twice the figure for boys as for girls and 83 per cent of the boys are in the 5–14 age group. Derangements of the knee joint number 565 and the peak with its male preponderance occurs after 15. Orthopaedic deformities numbered 2735. Except for these, which appear to be 'cold' cases, urgent or early admission is probably necessary to a unit in which relatively long stay is available as well as both orthopaedic and paediatric personnel.

A rheumatologist should also be in the team for the chronic rheumatoid conditions. These number 23 in the GP Morbidity Study, 10 being under the age of 5 years. The HIPE estimate is 631, with only 144 under 5 years. Extrapolation from the GP child population (1 in 167) gives a possible total of 3818. Comparison between these figures suggests that only a small proportion of affected children receives treatment in hospital and supports the views of rheumatologists that they are not being asked frequently enough to help in treatment and management of these extremely difficult children (Ansell 1975). This may well be an area where chronic disability extending into adult life might be diminished.

Class XIV. Congenital anomalies (ICD 740–759)

The health needs occasioned by congenital anomalies are included in the more general discussion on malformations in Chapter 5 and in particular contexts in Chapters 6, 9, 13, 14, 16, 17 and 18. The estimated discharges and deaths numbered 60 869 and RGSR records 3627 deaths. Of these 81 per cent occurred in the first year of life and 38 per cent within the first week.

Class XV. Certain causes of perinatal morbidity and mortality (ICD 760–779)

Comment on this class is especially difficult. The policy of hospital delivery rather than home confinement, whatever effects it may have on family life, does bring the fetus and the newborn baby into an area where experienced observation and technological aids are or should be available. That expert care is unevenly distributed throughout the population is unavoidable. Small maternity units inevitably lack experience of many of the relatively common problems of the perinatal period since the majority of deliveries are as normal as the babies that they produce and paediatric problems are absolutely rare.

The importance of the early diagnosis of the presence of congenital anomalies of the alimentary tract has already been discussed. The same holds true of cardio-vascular anomalies. The avoidance of respiratory difficulties and particularly of hypoxia is of such importance for the new baby's future, that special instruction should be given to all personnel, including the general practitioner, concerned with childbirth.

HIPE has 59 728 discharges and deaths in this class and RGSR, doubtless including some home confinements, records 6161 deaths. A quarter of the deaths, 1435 are of babies said to be immature, 24 947 (41.8 per cent of the class). Labelled 'anoxic and hypoxic *not elsewhere* classified' (ICD 776) are 11 505 estimated discharges and deaths, a group in which RGSR records 2537 deaths. Another 718 deaths are recorded for 'birth injury without mention of cause' (ICD 772) a group numbering 2491 in HIPE.

'Haemolytic disease with kernicterus' numbered 221 with 11 deaths and 'with no mention of kernicterus' 2580 with 185 deaths. In the data about stillbirth, haemolytic disease of the newborn is the listed cause of 338 deaths. In 19 there is said to have been no previous child, in 76 one, and in as many as 110 two previous children. Parity of three or more is recorded for another 108, and these figures suggest that modern methods of management are not being as widely used as they should be.

A large group of 'other conditions of fetus or newborn' numbers 11 638 and in this group there were 225 deaths.

The importance of the newborn period, which is well recognized, is not only assessed in relation to mortality, in which the figures are impressive enough. No less than one quarter of the total childhood deaths occur on the first day of life and by the end of the first week the percentage is above 40. Deaths under the age of one month were 9113 or 49 per cent of the total and by six months amounted to 12 688 or 68.5 per cent. What has to be remembered is that the amount of morbidity is also high at this period of rapid growth and development. The damage sustained as the result by those who survive illness must be taken into account in any assessment of child health needs.

Class XVI. Symptoms and ill-defined conditions (ICD 780–796)

This class is even less satisfactory than the others. A considerable use of hospital time and personnel is recorded, discharges from and deaths in hospital amounting to 68 143. It is fair to presume that accurate diagnosis was rarely achieved although a post-mortem examination was made in 91 per cent of the hospital sample in this Class. Only two serious conditions are recognizable, uraemia (22) and 'sudden death (cause unknown)' of which 1 is noted. There is, besides, the alarming but unrecognizable one called 'other ill-defined and unknown causes of morbidity and mortality' (4451). RGSR gives deaths from uraemia as 15, and from the ill-defined group as 25.

The RGSR deaths are recorded as 320. The largest number of deaths, 250, 75 per cent in the whole class is attributed to 'sudden death cause unknown', a number which includes sudden unexpected deaths when most of the babies die outside hospital. All but 30 died in the first six months of life. Deaths in this group in 1969 numbered 2, in 1970 51, in 1971 250, and in 1972 rose still further to 474, all but 78 under the age of six months. Coincidentally and despite the steady reduction in the number of live births, the groups 'homicide and purposely inflicted injury' and 'doubtful inflicted injuries' have not reduced, 91 and 38 respectively in 1970, 97 and 40 in 1971, and 105 and 31 in 1972.

There seem strong grounds for attempting to enhance methods of examination and for enlarging the data on which the cause of death is established when any baby dies under the age of six months. Perhaps some specialization for the examiners is needed. As practised today, dissection of the baby and histology do not discover the answer sufficiently often. Inclusion of social and psychological family background data might be revealing.

The only other groups in which deaths are noted are cardio-vascular and lymphatic, 1339 with 24 deaths, and general symptoms, 3924 with 5 deaths.

Of the non-fatal conditions, the largest number, 18 171, were admitted for abdominal symptoms aged 5 to 14 years, and 97 per cent of these for investigation of abdominal pain. Observation without need for further medical care accounted in the under fives for 11 892 and a further 6399 evenly divided between upper and lower gastro-intestinal tract. Under the heading 'Certain symptoms referable to nervous system and special senses' there were another 7950 of these young children.

In all, the under fives numbered 35 500 and the 5- to 14-year-olds 32 643. Perhaps a more effective use of out-patient facilities might have saved some of the children from admission. More effective use requires investigation departments and appointments services specifically aimed at economy in the use of hospital beds.

Class XVII. Accidents, poisonings and violence (ICD 800–999)

The health needs of children in relation to this serious and important class are more fully discussed in Chapter 19. The HIPE 1971 discharges and deaths are the second largest of all seventeen classes, 142 664, contributing 16.9 per cent of the total. In RGSR 1971, the 2122 deaths rank fourth with 11.4 per cent of the total. If deaths from the complications of childbirth and those due to congenital anomalies are omitted, this Class accounts for about one quarter of all childhood deaths in the total population. In the HIPE records, which refer only to the hospital population, the nature of the injury is the basis for the classification. The subgroups are:

fractures involving the skull and face (7253) with 544 deaths,
fractures and fracture dislocations (1074) with 98 deaths,
fractures of upper (12 634) with 3 deaths,
and of lower limbs (9622) with 4 deaths,
multiple fractures (310) with 7 deaths,
dislocations (1229) with 11 deaths,
sprains and strains (675) with no deaths,
concussion (9512) with 8 deaths,
intracranial injuries (36 795) with 192 deaths,
injuries to other organs (2458) with 241 deaths,
open wounds and amputations (9169) with 15 deaths,
superficial injuries and contusions (6267) with 2 deaths.

The other subgroups are foreign bodies (4628), burns (6777), nerve and spinal cord injuries (299), and adverse effects of medicinal (20 374) and toxic effects of non-medicinal substances (22 844). Together these groups account for 741 deaths, just over one third in the class (34.9 per cent). Unfortunately no less than 68.8 per cent of these (510) are classified as due to the effects of uncatalogued external causes other than extremes of temperature (0), radiation (0), air pressure (0), complications of surgical and medical care (3), early complications of trauma (2) and unspecified injury (5). Of the remaining 231 deaths, the largest single cause of death is carbon monoxide poisoning (120 or 51.9 per cent). To this number come contributions from 'fires and flames' and road traffic accidents.

Deaths from accidental falls numbered 135, 54 under the age of 3 years, and half of them (68) under the age of 5 years. Among accidents due to what are called natural and environmental factors (36), 29 are attributed to hunger, thirst, exposure and neglect, all but one in the first year and 23 in the first week of life. There were four suicides, all in the 10- to 14-year-old group. Homicide and inflicted injury, 97 in all, included 38 in the first year and there were 40 more, 16 in the first year, when such events as hanging, strangulation and drowning might have been purposeful.

Burns account for only 60 deaths, poisoning by medicinal substances for 27, only 9 of which relate to analgesics and antibiotics. Lead and its compounds including fumes account for 2 deaths.

When the question is availability of and expertise in treatment, the nature of the injury is more important than the nature of the accident. The use of hospital staff and departments is tailored to these needs. On the other hand, when the question of prevention is in issue, it is to the nature of the accident that attenion must be paid. RGSR (1971) gives very full details of deaths from accidents in the home and in residential institutions. These amounted to 557 in the 0- to 4-year age group and to 103 in the 5- to 14-year age group, a total of 660 or 31 per cent of all deaths attributable to accident. In a further 13 deaths the injury could have been purposely inflicted. The main single specified cause is 'inhalation and ingestion of food causing obstruction or suffocation' with 170 deaths of 0–4-year-olds and 4 of older children. 'Accidental mechanical suffocation in bed or cradle' accounted for another 92, all in the younger age group. Add to this the 93 deaths in this age group from accidents caused by fires and flames, and note that in 58 (62 per cent), despite the immense detail provided in the tables, the means remain unspecified. The need for serious research is clear.

There were 836 road traffic accidents, only 32 under the age of 2 but as many as 251 in the 10- to 14-year age group. Railway accidents (16) and water transport accidents (20) account for another 36 deaths.

HOSPITAL OUT-PATIENTS

Much of the most valuable preventive, therapeutic and supportive work is carried out by paediatricians in general paediatric out-patient clinics. Unfortunately there is as yet no systematic study of these activities. Specialist hospital clinics for the supervision of children with special diseases and disorders are referred to elsewhere in the text and an expected case-load can be estimated for some of these conditions. It would be both interesting and enlightening to mount an out-patient survey on the lines of the General Practice Survey in a few centres. The employment of trained medical receptionists with whom general practice secretaries could forge strong links might allow the saving of much time now occupied with waiting for consultations and for investigations. When such experienced people are available many of the patients can arrive for the medical consultation with much of the groundwork of diagnosis already done.

CHAPTER 11

The contribution of the general practitioner

One of the main purposes of the RCGP/BPA Project was to illuminate the part which the general practitioner should play in supplying the health needs of the children within the families in his practice. Only when the extent of his responsibility was known would it be possible to plan the nature and depth of his paediatric education.

Whether the primary care physician should remain a truly 'general practitioner' or whether he should specialize raises many questions and much may be said on both sides of the argument. Other countries have attempted solutions suitable to their populations. In the USA most of the primary care in the cities is delivered by paediatricians who do not normally see adults. By contrast the British family doctor, while he may have a special interest and that special interest may be child health, is expected to see patients of all age groups, an arrangement supported by the Royal College of General Practitioners. Nevertheless many practices carry out such work as prophylactic child health care and developmental assessment in special clinics run by only one or two members of the group. Other members would perhaps take on special clinics for ante- and post-natal care, family planning, cervical cytology or geriatrics.

Knowledge of current literature and special courses of instruction can keep the doctor with an interest au fait with developments in paediatrics. But for all doctors a basic knowledge of child care is essential, a requirement recognized by the paediatric content of the vocational training now planned for general practitioners. Because there are not enough available paediatric appointments, not every general practice vocational trainee will spend a full six months, but some paediatric training is provided in the general practice year. Knowledge of the total health needs of children should allow a more rational use to be made of this time.

The task of striking the balance between the kind and the amount of work to be done and the number of doctors available to provide the service, perhaps supplementing the numbers with non-medical personnel, is recognized as beyond the capability of the project. What needs to be done is described; to propose who is to do it is left to others.

Work with children will be done by many kinds of doctors as well as by those in general practice, both in the community and in hospital. The basic undergraduate training in paediatrics is essential for all. The content of the teaching programme could be tailored to some extent to meet the 'disease' demand, at least the commonly occurring conditions being covered. What has been called the quality in contrast to the quantity of the service demands an orientation of such teaching towards the seven facets of paediatrics discussed in Chapter 1. In addition there is the question of where the teaching should be conducted.

Disadvantages of hospital based paediatric teaching

Medical schools are traditionally based on hospitals. The whole paraphernalia of student selection, examination and certification would be difficult with any other sort of administrative structure. The advantages to all concerned, including the patients, are great. Nevertheless there are disadvantages which are the more serious for being often unperceived. The most important part of the hospital is the hospital bed and the most important person is not the patient in that bed but the consultant whose bed it is. Or was, for times are changing and much of hospital medicine is now practised by teams. Yet the teaching of medicine is orientated towards the kinds of disease for which admission into a hospital bed provides the solution, either because of the severity of the illness or of the technical demands of investigation or treatment. The attempt made here to quantify the medical health needs of children, if it does nothing else, shows how large are the health needs in the community itself and how limited is the number of sufferers from the conditions for which getting into bed in hospital is essential.

The comparison between the pattern of hospital morbidity and of what the population seeks from the general practitioner reveals striking differences. In the GP survey (Table 11.1) three groups of children form themselves – one contains the bulk of the work, in another the children with each diagnosis are fairly numerous and then there is a whole variety of conditions which are rarely seen. It may be that too little research and too little teaching are concerned with the first group, while the third, which includes many 'interesting cases', is researched and lectured about in medical schools. By the time the GP meets one of these rare conditions, he is likely to have completely forgotten what he was taught. The condition may not even have been recognized during his undergraduate courses.

Hospital paediatric practice teaches the need for precision in diagnosis and the importance of homeostasis. It also illustrates the value of explanation and support for parents who are now more and more involved in the care of their hospitalized offspring. That hospital teaching is not

Table 11.1 Total numbers of general practitioner consultations in thousands and percentage of total in each class
From GPR, 1971. Table 11 (ICD classification 1965)

		Thousands	*Per cent of total*
VIII	Diseases of the respiratory system (460–519)	38.6	32.5
XVI	Symptoms and ill-defined conditions (780–796)	13.3	11.2
XVIII	Prophylactic procedures and other medical examinations (Y06-0-61)	12.8	10.7
VI	Diseases of the nervous system and sense organs (320–389)	12.6	10.6
I	Infective and parasitic diseases (000–136)	11.8	9.9
XII	Diseases of the skin and sub-cutaneous tissue (680–709)	11.2	9.4
XVII	Accidents, poisonings and violence (800–999, Y60–79)	7.0	5.9
V	Mental disorders (290–315)	3.1	2.6
IX	Diseases of the digestive tract (520–577)	3.0	2.5
X	Diseases of genito-urinary system (580–629)	2.1	1.7
XIII	Diseases of the musculo-skeletal system and connective tissue (710–738)	1.3	1.0
XIV	Congenital anomalies (740–759)	0.5	0.4
III	Endocrine, nutritional and metabolic diseases (240–279)	0.4	0.3
IV	Diseases of blood and blood forming organs (280–289)	0.4	0.3
II	Neoplasms (140–239)	0.2	0.16
VII	Diseases of circulatory system (390–458)	0.2	0.16
XV	Certain causes of perinatal mortality and morbidity (760–779)	0.1	0.08
XI	Complications of pregnancy, childbirth and the puerperium (630–678)	0.016	—
	Total	118.6	99.4

enough is well recognized and in many medical schools the student receives part of his paediatric education in the community.

Another important change is the introduction of lectures early in the course on physical, intellectual and emotional growth and development, which will contribute to the better future provision for child health needs by showing more clearly their true nature. Traditional teaching begins with the mature adult as if he was never a fetus in the womb who has passed through perinatal dangers, childhood's stresses and adolescent temptations to become the man that he is. The developmental concept holds a key place in paediatrics.

The general practitioner as a family doctor

The general practitioner, as the primary care doctor, must be able to recognize the conditions and the situations demanding hospital care and management. Hospital out-patient departments need to be better organized so that they may adequately serve as diagnostic and special supervision centres with the minimum of delay and the maximum of co-operation. But it is the non-hospital matters that should mainly occupy his attention and his interest. What can be safely managed in the home must differ between village and city and between social classes, and decisions will be more accurately made the better known the family is to its medical adviser. The paternalistic 'village doctor' still exists and he can even survive within the mass population of a city. The chances of his survival vary inversely with the demand for medical services. The results of overstraining practices are seen in fragmented care with a rota of duty hours. At least two factors are likely to increase demand. Health education and the publication of medical knowledge through the media spread information about disease rather than health and about treatment rather than prevention. The second factor is the taxation, direct and indirect, of the individual to pay for the free National Health Service. As he pays for it he might as well use it. He attracts no further cost. The habit of the members of one family to register with different practices must also diminish the personal involvement of one doctor in the medical affairs of an individual family.

This would matter less were the doctor's main duty the primary care of acute physical illness, the treatment of infections or the recognition of surgical emergencies. Essential though these services are, the study of stress and its effects on health has pointed directly towards the importance of interpersonal relationships. In paediatrics the focus of these relationships is the family. It becomes increasingly difficult to treat one member of a family in isolation. To the fundamental idea of development as the most important general one in paediatrics must be added the absolute importance of intra-familial relationships. Full development of potential is only possible within the context of adequate family life.

The traditional western doctor is the personal physician. A later arrival has been the physician concerned with the public health. What is now being studied and illuminated is the health of the family, not as a collection of individuals who happen to live at the same address, but as a unit with its own diseases and disorders and its own psychopathology. The formula that 'the Englishman's home is his castle' has been accompanied by the unspoken belief that what happens within that home is 'this Englishman's business'. That this may be no longer acceptable is suggested by the growing interest in the drafting of a 'Bill of Rights for Children'. Child health needs include love and security among many other things which can only be provided within the family. A society that is truly concerned with the mental and physical health of its children must examine from this family point of view the effects of its social legislation, its policies for housing, wages and employment, together with its moral attitudes. What is likely to happen to the deprived child is now predictable. The family-less child is the one who suffers from the greatest deprivation of all.

This is not to say that the effects of the stress of deprivation are bound always to be harmful. The child who can adjust to serious stress may benefit in maturity, independence and insight. Perhaps the comparison with the effects of severe infective disease in early life may be just. When epidemics of infantile diarrhoea and vomiting produced a high infant mortality rate, those who did survive proved to be wonderfully healthy and long-lived. Excessive emotional stress does not often kill and sometimes strengthens, but it is more likely to leave a personality damaged for life.

At present there is being added to the personal physician and his public health colleagues, a third figure, overshadowing the latter, the community physician. His main angle of vision is likely to be the family viewed from the state, society and other families. What is suggested here is the development of a general practitioner who studies the family, not so much from the outside as from within. Child health centres and practices serve 'good' patients and 'bad'. The former come when they should, listen to, understand and carry out instructions, the 'bad' ones do none of these things. In reality the 'good' could manage most of their health affairs without outside help at all. But whereas they may not need the doctor, the doctor – like the health visitor – needs them to provide that feeling of well-being, of usefulness, of success so necessary to the provider of the service and afforded only by the satisfied client. To intervene when unwanted, to educate, to support the 'bad' patients and so to prevent mental ill-health, may be one of the most important functions of the paediatric community physician. He will need to know how to recognize the depriving family and how to get his foot in the door so as to overcome the effect of deprivations which include depriving the child of medical care and the family of much needed support.

This general discussion provides a background for the more detailed discussion of the morbidity statistics and suggests some of the obstacles that block the doctor's view of the realities of the patient's situation. The diagnostic labels are after all no more than the nearest possible approximations offered by a diagnostic classification. In practice they enable the doctor to extract from the patient's total situation those elements that are suitable for 'medical' treatment. Not to notice the rest is all too easy.

Morbidity statistics from general practice

As with all medical statistics the basis of the GP survey is the international classification of disease and no other basis seems possible. Some comment about the quality of medical practice may place the ICD data in a perspective of people rather than of labels. For the description of medical work categorized in this way must suffer more or less distortion in order to make it fit. The apparently simple question to the patient 'Why did you send for me/come to see me?' cannot be given a simple answer. Even were the doctor only the diagnoser of acute infective disease and the prescriber of the correct antibiotic, such problems as pain, sleep, fear, anxiety, loss of confidence remain.

Rehabilitation after accident needs as much understanding of family and personal characteristics as do chronic school problems, failure to live up to parental expectations and delayed maturity. Family situations donning the cloak of symptoms disguise themselves as diseases. One entry under ICD No. 785 covering flatulence, colic, appendicular and other non-colicky pain may be no more than the presenting tip of a matrimonial and domestic iceberg. The pastoral care of a family with a handicapped child, whether physically or mentally, is discussed in Chapter 9. Everything depends on the role which the doctor accepts as his.

The survey involved 53 practices and 118 doctors serving a population of 191 247 containing 69 748 children, or 1 in 167 of the total child population. The under-5-year-olds numbered 21 600, the over-fives 48 148.

More than 84 per cent of all patients consulting about children (Table 11.1) came from six diagnostic classes, respiratory (VIII) 32.5 per cent, ill-defined (XVI) 11.2 per cent, central nervous system and sense organs (VI) 10.6 per cent, infective and parasitic diseases (I) 9.9 per cent, skin diseases (XII) 9.5 per cent. The third largest class (XVIII) comprises prophylactic procedures and other medical examinations (10.7 per cent). Accidents, poisonings and violence (XVII) provide 5.9 per cent, the digestive tract (IX) 2.6 per cent, mental disorders (V) 2.6 per cent, genito-urinary tract (X) 1.8 per cent and musculo-skeletal (XIII) 1.1 per cent. The remaining seven classes together contribute less than 2 per cent and these include such important and serious conditions as neoplasms, endocrine and metabolic disorders, diseases of the blood and blood-forming organs, of the heart and circulation, congenital defects, perinatal disorders and disorders of childbirth. Patients in these classes can be utilized for much clinical teaching and their disorders fit excellently into lectures as well as into examination questions.

The order of frequency for the under-5-year-olds and the 5-year-old-and-older children does not differ materially. As expected prophylactic injections and health education bring the Class XVIII for under-fives up from third to second place when compared with the whole group, but it constitutes only 17.3 per cent of the work load for the younger age group.

The following comments relate to the 18 diagnostic classes.

Class I, infective and parasitic diseases, is the fifth largest group, with 11 791 patients consulting and forming 10.9 per cent of the total. As already noted in Chapter 10, many more patients suffering from the effects of infection are to be found in other classes. For example there were more patients consulting for naso-pharyngitis (Class VIII, 14 560) than are included in the whole of Class I. About one in five of the children in Class I had some form of diarrhoea and/or vomiting. Winter vomiting disease (238, or 2 per cent) is listed separately.

The acute specific fevers provided 42.9 per cent (5 057) and their needs would have been establishing a diagnosis for the first affected child in the family, helping to plan quarantine or isolation and notification when appropriate. No doubt many children, unprotected by immunization, pass through these illnesses without benefit of doctor. In the year of the Survey (1970-71) measles provided one quarter of the fevers (1359) a number due to diminish appreciably with the success of the immunization programme. Rubella contributed 23 per cent (1178), chickenpox 21.5 per cent (1089), whooping cough 11.3 per cent (572), mumps 7.9 per cent (401) and streptococcal sore throat and scarlet fever 7.1 per cent (359).

Probably greater diagnostic problems were presented by infectious mononucleosis (105) and infective hepatitis (99). More serious infections were meningococcal 11, acute poliomyelitis (surprisingly) 3, herpes zoster 118, Bornholm disease 6, and aseptic meningitis 31.

Among the fringe conditions in which parental tolerance plays an important part in determining their recognition, supplemented by the activity of the educational welfare officer for children at school, are scabies and pediculosis, 453 and 88, contributing 10.7 per cent. As to intestinal parasites, a population survey would be expected to show, by perianal swab techniques, that between 30 and 40 per cent of children carry oxyuris, some 25 000 among the children in the survey. In fact in the practices survey only 258 children presented for treatment and no means exist for telling on what the diagnosis was based. Other intestinal helminthiasis was diagnosed in 226, the whole group contributing 9.5 per cent. Incompletely diagnosed patients (85) and those diagnosed but not separately listed (624) accounted for 14.0 per cent. Moniliasis is presumably included among diagnoses not separately listed in the report.

As a gentle reminder of past times, 13 children consulted for some form of tuberculous infection and 2 for venereal disease.

On the whole, the patients in this class should not have taxed either the diagnostic or the therapeutic expertise of the doctors, whose general training should have familiarized them with these illnesses without any deep penetration into paediatrics. Indeed parents themselves are often able to make the correct diagnosis as readily as the doctor.

Class II, neoplasms, is small with 186 consultations (0.15 per cent), only 7 malignant with 2 children suffering from leukaemia. Of the remaining benign neoplasms, 177, the skin was involved in 92. This does not include haemangiomas, whose whereabouts cannot be identified. There were 20 consultations for benign neoplasms of the breast, 11 in males. The term neoplasm may or may not be preferable to the older term mastitis as a description of a normal stage in development, yet this illustrates a general deficiency in the classification. Many normal developmental processes, presenting with symptoms or physical signs, lead to medical consultations and at times to unnecessary medical and surgical activities. Such consultations cannot be fitted accurately into the list. The placing of a little girl on a waiting list for biopsy is not unknown when one breast develops before the other. There is too the anxiety lest a child might have leukaemia, especially after leukaemia publicity, a most important consultation for the relief of family anxiety.

Class III, endocrine, nutritional and metabolic diseases, is also small, with 387 consultations (0.3 per cent). The largest entry is for obesity (242, 62.5 per cent). Avitaminoses and other nutritional disorders contribute 38, diabetes mellitus 29 and there were 17 consultations for thyroid disturbances including 7 cretins. Although small in numbers, this class requires much servicing including supervision of diet and of prescribed treatment. The difficulties in the successful treatment of obesity have been discussed in Chapter 4, and the management of children with diabetes mellitus in Chapter 17.

Class IV, diseases of blood and blood-forming organs, represents 0.3 per cent of consultations (393). One diagnosis, in this case iron-deficiency anaemia, provides two thirds of the consultations (66.6 per cent). Somewhat unexpectedly these are common in the 5-year-old and over group, 166, with 96 in the under-fives. The criteria for diagnosis are, of course, not revealed. If this represents a true deficiency of iron and if results from these practices can be fairly extrapolated to the general population, some educational effort over diet or some screening examination of younger children might repay the expenditure of time and money. Purpura and haemorrhagic conditions account for 38 and among the rest are 9 diagnosed pernicious anaemia, 6 of them under the age of 5 years.

Class V, mental disorders, includes 2.6 per cent (3089) of all consultations and raises questions of the authenticity of diagnoses. Various forms of neurosis amount to 439 (14.2 per cent) the two main types being anxiety (250) and depressive (101). 64 of the 439 (14.4 per cent) are children under five. Psychosis is rarely diagnosed (17) but there is a large number (1209, 39 per cent) labelled 'special symptoms not elsewhere classified, transitory situational disturbances and child behaviour disturbances'. Mental retardation contributes 47 (1.5 per cent). Physical disorders of presumably psychogenic origin number 323 (10.4 per cent). There is no recognizable group where psychological disorders are blamed on physical disease, but these consultations are probably included under other headings. There can be no denying that they exist or that parents consult about them with their general practitioners.

Two other diagnoses deserve comment. Insomnia, that might be better named sleep disturbance, contributes 356 (11.5 per cent). About 4 out of 5 of these are for the under-5-year-olds. Experience would suggest that the main prevalence is in the age period 6 to 24 months and that the doctor is only one of many called upon to advise about management. The other diagnosis is enuresis and once more criteria of diagnosis need discussion. Parents exist who consult the doctor because their 2- or 3-year-old child still wets the bed. Of the 587 consultations (19.0 per cent) no less than 114, one in five, were for children in the younger age group, when many doctors would regard continued bed-wetting as usually normal (see p. 186). Both insomnia and enuresis in children are in the main developmental rather than mental disorders. Support could be mobilized for making three sub-divisions in this class, mental retardation, neurosis and psychosis, and behaviour disturbances which represent difficulties in development. For the first, full assessment and specialized help in management are essential. The second need psychiatric care. For the third and largest the general practitioner should have sufficient understanding following sufficient training to be able to treat most families. Insofar as he needs help in diagnosis and continuing care, he should be able to find it, for the younger child in the child health centre and for all children in his neighbourhood paediatric clinic.

Class VI, diseases of the nervous system and sense organs, with a total of 12 636 consultations (10.8 per cent), is made up of three sections. Nervous diseases as listed account for 451 (0.4 per cent), diseases involving the 'eye', using this word in a very loose sense to include the conjunctiva, the lids and the eye muscles, 4096 (3.4 per cent), and of the ear, 8089 (6.8 per cent).

The main component of the *nervous system diseases* is migraine (213, 47.2 per cent) largely in the 5-year-old and over group, and the next is epilepsy (167, 37.0 per cent). Once more the criteria for definitive diagnosis come into question. What differentiates headache from migraine in childhood and at what point do seizures earn the title of epilepsy? The really difficult diagnoses of degenerative diseases are concealed within the 33 labelled 'other diseases of the central nervous system (including hereditary and familial)' and the 23 labelled 'other diseases of the nervous system'.

The management of the child with epilepsy is discussed in Chapter 14 with that of the child with cerebral palsy, and the general topic of mental handicap in Chapter 13. Psychiatric disturbances are considered in Chapter 12. The responsibilities of the general practitioner form part of each discussion.

The *eye diseases* are chiefly infective. Conjunctivitis (2268), blepharitis (337), hordeolum (369), and inflammation of the lacrymal apparatus (83) total 74.6 per cent (3057), and on the whole do not require any deep acquaintance with either ophthalmology or paediatrics. On the other hand such relatively common conditions should form the subject for teaching as should the early recognition and management of strabismus (288, 7.0 per cent) and refractive errors (424, 10.3 per cent). 'Other diseases of the eye' (230, 5.6 per cent) probably include many for whom ophthalmologist's help was required.

The *ear* provides the largest number (8089, 6.4 per cent). As with the eye, the main problem is infection, acute otitis media contributing 6467 (79.9 per cent), chronic otitis media 162 (2.0 per cent) and mastoiditis a further 7, a total of 6636 consultations (82.0 per cent). 'Other diseases of the ear and mastoid process' (232), and otosclerosis (3) contibute 2.9 per cent, who would be likely to need specialist attention, while otitis externa (421) and wax in the ear (531) totalling 11.7 per cent, would certainly not. 'Other deafness' accounts for 257 (3.1 per cent). It is an interesting reflection of the medical and even the paediatric outlook of the past that while the organs of sight and hearing are categorized in some detail, no space is allowed for disorders of speech and communication presumably because the doctor is not regarded as either diagnostician or therapist.

Class VII, diseases of the circulatory system, is one of the three least common with only 165 consultations (0.1 per cent). When chilblains (49), haemorrhoids (14) and varicose veins (4) are subtracted, together with other named and unnamed diseases of the circulation, only 61 consultations remain for acquired diseases of the heart. The commonest is rheumatic heart disease (11), and then disorders of rhythm (10), cardiomyopathy (7), and congestive heart failure (4) with 'other and ill-defined heart disease' (13). Congenital heart and circulatory disease is included under congenital anomalies in Class XIV. Doubtful heart sounds and murmurs and their place in the computations are referred to in Chapter 16. The rarity of these conditions in any one practice would make the use of specialist services advisable. The finding of chilblains in this class raises the question of which department in the medical school has the responsibility for teaching about this condition.

Class VIII, diseases of respiratory system, is responsible for almost one third of all consultations (38 583, 32.5 per cent). Much medical time is consumed in the diagnosis and many prescriptions in the treatment of these conditions, although not every child with respiratory symptoms is taken to a doctor. The subject is full of mysteries and unsolved problems. The availability of chest x-rays has added its quota of both expense and mystery.

Acute infections of the upper respiratory tract account for over two thirds of the consultations (27 172, 70.4 per cent). Acute bronchitis (5912) and influenza (310) for a further 16.1 per cent (6222). Pleurisy (11), pleural effusion (6), bronchiectasis (9) and pneumothorax (4), provide little work for the general practitioner. As to pneumonia, there were 125 consultations in the older age group and 103 in the under-fives, but this includes pneumonia of the newborn which is a different kind of disease in most cases and is rarely due to bacterial or virus infection.

The allergic conditions of the respiratory tract number asthma 1048, emphysema 1, hay fever 953 and possibly chronic bronchitis 101, a total of 2103 (5.4 per cent). The difficulties of assessing the part played by allergic responses in what resemble acute respiratory infections in children, especially the under-fives, are discussed in Chapter 16. There is room for research and teaching in this important area. The studies of respiratory syncytial virus infection and its effects in the early months of life should shed light on these correlations.

Two other headings, catarrh and hypertrophy of tonsils and adenoids, need defining. Both are numerically important, catarrh with 1905 consultations (4.9 per cent of the class) and hypertrophy of tonsils and adenoids with 375 (1.0 per cent). The latter diagnosis was made in 104 children under the age of 5 years, when the tonsils are expected to be at their largest. The criteria for recognizing such hypertrophy must indeed be difficult to establish (see Chapter 16).

Objectivity is hard to achieve for the patients and the conditions in this class. In life the acute infections are seasonal and epidemic and therefore the doctor of primary care is rushed off his feet and exhausted by calls at just the time when a cool head and a detailed observation of the patient might well allow some of the questions to be answered. The logical approach to teaching must await these answers. Meanwhile practice depends upon general principles, habit of mind and prejudice.

Class IX, diseases of digestive system, contributes 3081 consultations (2.6 per cent). Of these 1320 belong to the dental department and there remain 2761. The largest single group is constipation (487, 17.5 per cent), followed by hernia, femoral and inguinal (222, 8.0 per cent) and appendicitis (181, 6.5 per cent). Among smaller listed groups are peptic ulcer (13), disease of liver and gall bladder (12), and anal fissure (58). The second largest group is called disorders of function of stomach (231). The classification gives little indication of the importance of the alimentary tract in paediatrics. Acute infective gastro-enteritis has already been encountered in Class I and Class XVI in its turn will reveal a large number of consultations about symptoms referable to this tract. A scientific study of the diseases and disorders of the alimentary system would need as a first step a careful definition of terms used. Chronic constipation may mean no more than the daily passing of a hard stool but it may mean refusal to defaecate resulting in one stool a fortnight. Ideas of treatment vary as widely as does the philosophy behind the treatment. Further discussion, especially about abdominal pain, will be found in Chapter 16 as well as later in this chapter (Class XVI).

Class X, diseases of genito-urinary system, is another small group with 2106 consultations (1.8 per cent) and once more infection contributes the greater number. Pyelitis, pyelonephritis, pyelocystitis (234), cystitis (acute 532 and chronic 20), account for 37.3 per cent (786). Nephritis and nephrosis (12) and renal calculus (13) are rare. Urethritis was diagnosed in 40 and 'other disease of urinary tract' in 92. How far were cultures of adequately collected urine specimens the basis for the diagnosis of urinary infections? Because of the implications of prolonged drug treatment and the possibility that inadequate treatment may damage the kidneys, this is an important subject for teaching. Errors are easily made in over as well as under diagnosis.

Diseases of the male genitalia are hydrocele (36), orchitis and epididymitis (12) and 'other diseases' (649), a total of 697 (33.0 per cent of the class). The 'other diseases' include redundant prepuce and phimosis. Diseases of the female genital tract amount to 350 (16.7 per cent), 216 are concerned with menstruation, 117 with non-venereal vaginal discharge and 65 are labelled 'other diseases of female genitalia'. There were 56 consultations about diseases of the breast, 24 in boys and 32 in girls. The diagnosis excludes neoplasm but includes cysts (see p. 116).

Class XI, complications of pregnancy, childbirth and the puerperium, is expectedly the smallest class with only 16 consultations. The question of precocious sexual activity is discussed in Chapter 10 and it is of interest to find in the survey practices that there were 12 normal pregnancies in girls under the age of 15 years, 10 pregnancies with complications and 6 abortions, only 1 of which was spontaneous.

Class XII, diseases of the skin and subcutaneous tissue, is the fifth largest cause for consultation (11 264, 9.5 per cent) and this suggests the need for sound basic training in paediatric dermatology. It is true that infections of these tissues contribute 41.1 per cent (4634), 35 per cent of them diagnosed as impetigo (1634). Eczema and dermatitis, not differentiated, amount to 32.5 per cent (3656). Infantile eczema is included with non-allergic and unspecified skin conditions in the largest single group (2638 with 1528 under 5). Named skin diseases number 958 with another 967 labelled urticaria. Acne vulgaris brought 323 five years old and over to consultation. Pruritus (213), corns and callosities (59), diseases of the nail (133), of hair and hair follicles (120), of sweat and sebaceous glands (147) and pigmentation (10) swell the total. There remain 347 diagnosed as 'other signs, symptoms and incompletely diagnosed conditions in this group'.

Class XIII, diseases of the musculo-skeletal system and connective tissue, contribute 1291 (1.1 per cent). Four elements compose this class, rheumatoid and osteo-arthritic conditions (215, 16.6 per cent), the results of injury and strain (420, 32.5 per cent), deformities, flat foot and hallux valgus and varus (173, 13.4 per cent), and 'other diseases of musculo-skeletal and connective tissue' (485, 37.5 per cent). These diseases produce both pain and disability, the latter possibly life-long. The availability of paediatric orthopaedic clinics for assessment, treatment plans, supervision and in some areas actual treatment facilities would seem essential. Rheumatoid arthritis in particular is discussed on page 102.

Class XIV, congenital anomalies, is a surprisingly small group, numbering only 483 (0.4 per cent). This may be because the services of the general practitioner are by-passed and the treatment and supervision of affected children are undertaken by the hospital service. This is understandable in the case of spina bifida, meningo-myelocele and hydrocephalus where a number of specialists is inevitably involved. Consultations for these conditions are recorded as 34 (7.0 per cent). The heart and circulation account for 73 (15.1 per cent), cleft palate and hare lip 9 (1.8 per cent), congenital anomaly of the digestive system 19 (3.9 per cent), of the genito-urinary system 51 (10.5 per cent), of bone and joint 120 (24.8 per cent), of other specified kinds not listed separately 108 (22.3 per cent) and an imprecisely defined group of 68 (14.0 per cent). Except for babies born at home, the likelihood is that case finding and diagnosis would be the responsibility of the hospital. It could be that, apart from the care of acute illness in those affected, the general practitioner could make a greater contribution than he does to morale support for the family and to help in adjusting the home environment to the needs of the handicapped child (see Chapter 9).

Class XV, certain causes of perinatal morbidity and mortality, with 109 consultations (0.1 per cent) cannot be discussed in detail since 67 (61.4 per cent) are grouped together as 'other causes of perinatal morbidity'. The diagnosis of immaturity accounts for 19 and of haemolytic disease for 12. If obstetrics is regarded as a part of hospital practice, the general practitioner is unlikely to be in a position to provide a neonatal medical service. While he must be well acquainted with fetal and neonatal physiology and anatomy and with the examination and the recognition of the normality of these special forms of human being, it is doubtful how deeply the routine undergraduate general teaching need delve into neonatology.

Class XVI, symptoms and ill-defined conditions, is the second largest with 13 384 consultations (12.66 per cent). The categories are avowedly the titles of symptoms and physical signs and form an interesting supplement to the other classes which are system based. Either occasion or opportunity was lacking for further study of the patient by the general practitioner and some would doubtless have been sent on for consultant opinion. The general pattern of frequency is repeated with cough providing the largest single category (4168 or 31.1 per cent) with a further group of respiratory tract problems (454) giving a total of 4622 (34.5 per cent of this class) as a supplement to Class VIII. There were 286 consultations for epistaxis. Of alimentary tract disorders, 3612 are for acute vomiting and/or diarrhoea and the next largest group consists of various forms of abdominal pain (716). The supplement to Class IX (digestive tract) amounts to 1840 (13.7 per cent of this class). The genito-urinary system contributes 419 (3.1 per cent), irregularities of micturition numbering 211. The main reason for consultation in diseases of the central nervous system (340, 2.5 per cent) is convulsions with 107, the next being vertigo (56). The 'other symptoms, etc' group is 142.

Referable to the heart and circulation are 108 (0.8 per cent) with 68 diagnosed syncope. One large group involved skin rashes, (without pyrexia 995, and with pyrexia 206, a total of 1201, 8.9 per cent). Fever alone amounted to 568 (4.2 per cent). Another group of 'other symptoms, signs and incompletely diagnosed conditions' accounted for 786 consultations (5.8 per cent).

This class gives possibly the best insight into the dilemmas with which the general practitioner is faced in making his decision on the need to investigate a problem further. General practice experience added to natural clinical aptitude seem to be what he needs rather than any didactic teaching.

Class XVII, accidents, poisonings and violence, makes a surprisingly small contribution (7077, 5.9 per cent) unless for the pattern of a pyramid with the top layers going to hospital is substituted an explosion. In the centre are the severe hospital emergency cases and at the periphery those treatable at home or school without a doctor's help. The doctor is called in in the relatively small area between. This concept is borne out by the distribution of the injuries the largest group being soft tissue injuries (2623, 51.2 per cent) and one of the smallest internal injuries (11). Again sprains and strains account for 20.1 per cent (1283) while fractures for only 6.3 per cent (451). Insect bites number 528 (7.5 per cent). The total of burns is 285 (4.0 per cent) only 13 of third degree while foreign bodies entering into orifices number 158 (1.1 per cent), the normal lay reaction being to rush to hospital with severe burns and foreign body problems.

Poisoning too is rare, 4 from aspirin, 3 from barbiturates and 115 others seen in one year in 53 practices. A group of 'other injuries and effects of external causes' accounts for another 1.9 per cent (211).

Class XVIII, prophylactic procedures and other medical examinations, amount to 12 787 (10.7 per cent). Here the general practitioner plays his invaluable part in health education and preventive medicine. The largest group comprises routine immunization, vaccination against smallpox and immunization under special circumstances against the acute specific fevers (7607, 59.5 per cent). To this may be added immunization against the typhoid group and cholera (432, 3.4 per cent). Routine and other medical examinations account for 2694 consultations (21 per cent) mainly in the under-fives (2067) and presumably most in the first year.

Prenatal and postnatal care (15), oral contraceptive advice (18) and other contraceptive advice (5) for boys as well as girls under 15 years old reflects the modern fashion in sexual behaviour.

Health education and instruction amount to 1747 (13.6 per cent).

Conclusion

This discussion of the work of the general practitioner with children, obviously superficial though it be, shows that the bulk of his paediatric practice concerns very different matters from those seen by hospital-based paediatricians. His role is to be at hand, available to help in the primary care of acute illness, usually of infective origin and most commonly involving the upper and lower respiratory tracts. The volume of morbidity is large albeit that most is of 'minor' or self-limiting illness. Hidden within this mass are serious, even life-endangering conditions whose recognition demands constant vigilance. He must find for the presenting symptoms and signs the appropriate steps – reassurance, relief, or referral for specialist consultation. Next in quantity comes his work in active prevention or health education. Here he can use the relationship formed through the care of illness to watch over the child's growth and development within the family. After this come diseases, again mostly infective, of ear, eye, skin and subcutaneous tissues and the diagnosis and treatment of certain special infections and infestations. Lastly he contributes to the management of the results of accidents, poisonings and violence. The part that he plays in psychiatric and mental disease is small, but emotional and psychological disturbance in their own right make heavy demands on time. Unmeasured and unmeasurable is what he accomplishes in relation to the family anxieties and tensions that surround illness. The fact of his existence in the neighbourhood, available to help when called upon, a reliable establishment figure to whom all his patients can relate, is by no means the least of his achievements. He is a necessary provider of peace of mind about health and disease in Western society.

Many general practitioners have already accepted their role in those aspects of paediatrics described in Chapter 1 other than the immediate treatment of disease. The altered pattern of illness in the community has been accompanied by an altered and wider approach to aetiology and to management, much of which is included in social and community medicine. If the general practitioner is expected to understand environmental factors including emotional stress in aetiology and the comprehensive nature of management, bringing in as it must the work of other professionals and if his standards are to be securely based on a knowledge of the normal child and the normal growth and development of mind, body and emotional maturity, the question arises of where he is to learn and to gain this experience. The hospital can provide the base but he will need surely to move out into the community. Only when teaching in the community supplements teaching in the ward and the laboratory can the course be completed.

CHAPTER 12

Psychiatric disorders

A study of the health needs of children would indeed be incomplete, which paid no attention to emotional disturbance, maladjustment and patterns of behaviour regarded as abnormal because unacceptable to parents, teachers or society. On the other hand, no satisfactory classification exists within the framework of which a realistic assessment of quantity can be fitted. To number all the children by year of age who wet the bed, dirty their pants, bite their nails or have nightmares or recurrent abdominal pain adds but little to the sum of human knowledge; Douglas has shown that 11-year-olds with these symptoms tend to be educationally handicapped in many ways (Douglas *et al.* 1968). But it does not of itself provide a guide to the number of children whose condition demands treatment from a psychiatrist, a paediatrician or a general practitioner. The problem is that the quality of the behaviour is not critical, it is rather its quantity, its persistence and the tolerance of those against whom it appears to be directed and who feel threatened by it. Parents and teachers eventually turn in desperation to therapeutic experts for help. The character of the symptoms determines the direction in which they go for advice. The point in time at which they acknowledge their desperation depends on, among many factors, the availability of services, so that the demand must always outstrip the supply. Fortunately, children can grow through these problems, and the great majority of those who would feature on the list suggested above of the wet, the dirty and the rest, discard their symptoms as time passes, and their names come off the treatment waiting list. To what extent they are strengthened, to what extent damaged by the experience, is unknown.

Some data are available in the classical surveys, of Douglas, Newcastle. Isle of Wight, and the National Children's Bureau and in gross numbers in statistical reports from the DES. In drawing conclusions from these observations and applying them to the total child population, attention must always be paid to both the purpose of and the philosophy underlying the collection of the figures, a general discussion of which appears in Chapter 2.

Classification

Rutter, for the Isle of Wight study, devised a pragmatic classification of psychiatric disorder into seven groups:

1 Neurotic: abnormality of the emotions with no loss of reality sense, e.g. anxiety, depression, obsession, compulsion, phobia, hypochondriasis, conversion hysteria.
2 Antisocial or conduct: behaviour giving rise to social disapproval, e.g. delinquency, bullying, destructiveness, fixed sexual perversion.
3 Mixed conduct and neurotic: nearer anti-social than neurotic.
4 Hyperkinetic syndrome: poorly organized or regulated activity, distractibility, short attention span, impulsiveness, fluctuation of mood not secondary to psychiatric disturbance.
5 Childhood psychosis: infant; later regressive and disintegrative; speech involvement as in elective mutism; schizophrenia; manic-depressive.
6 Other, which are not included with 1 to 5.
7 Developmental disorder covered by specific delays in biological maturation which were not secondary to another psychiatric syndrome. In practice this means enuresis and in later surveys the seventh group is treated separately as are disorders of speech, language and fine manipulation (Rutter *et al*. 1970).

Prevalence

A point prevalence at 10 and 11 years was estimated from an elaborate questionnaire for the 2199 children of those ages in the Isle of Wight study. The corrected rate for the seven categories was 6.8 per cent (Rutter *et al.* 1970). Excluded were children with mono-symptomatic disorders and with uncomplicated intellectual or educational retardation. The largest groups were neurotic disorders (2.5 per cent) mainly anxiety, and conduct taken together with mixed conduct and neurotic disorders (4.0 per cent). There were only 3 per thousand in the remaining four categories. Two children were classed as hyperkinetic, two as psychotic and 'one girl had a markedly deviant personality'.

Applied to the 1971 population at 10 and 11 years ($n = 1\,521\,300$), assuming an even spread, the expected numbers for England and Wales would be 38 032 children with neurotic disorders and 60 852 with conduct and mixed conduct and neurotic disorders. The total number with psychiatric disturbance would have been 103 448. Among the Isle of Wight children only fifteen, one in ten of those identified as having a psychiatric disorder, were under psychiatric treatment, an estimated 10 350 in the 1971 10- and 11-year-old group.

Of practical importance is the finding that children with physical disorders showed significantly more neurotic and anti-social disorders than the general child population, asthmatic children twice as frequently and those with epilepsy and neurological disorders three or four times as frequently. There was, besides, a correlation between reading retardation and anti-social behaviour, both possibly developing on the basis of similar types of temperamental deviance. Delinquency may itself arise in response to educational failure.

The Newcastle prediction of expected disabilities for every 5000 children entering school is 200 with behaviour disorders (Miller *et al.* 1960), a point prevalence at 5 years of 4.0 per cent, recognized by the observers as probably an under-estimate, but one that would yield 32 000 among the 1971 school entrants. Information came, not from questionnaire, but from parental discussions with health visitors, few having sought medical advice.

In the National Children's Bureau Cohort at seven years of age studied by questionnaire, behaviour and adjustment were related to differences in sex, social class and region, a cut-off point in scoring being used that left 6 per cent for study. The accent was on prevention in the future rather than on prevalence now.

Howells (1972) has analyzed one thousand cases of 0 to 19 years at the Children's Intake Clinic, the Institute of Family Psychiatry, the Ipswich Hospital. Only 6 (0.6 per cent) were psychotic, a proportion similar to Rutter's figure of those who required psychiatric treatment. Howells regarded the rest (99.4 per cent) as emotionally disturbed as the result of family stress.

He quotes a Danish survey of all children up to 15 years old on Samsö Island where 15.5 per cent needed psychiatric care. 'Statisticians estimate this as equivalent to 2–3 per cent of children needing care per year . . .' This would produce between 233 500 and 350 300 in the 1971 Project group, so that about 30 000 would be in need of psychiatric treatment (1 in 10) in any one year.

A review of these studies suggests that growing up, which includes adjusting to life in a growing family and attending school in order to receive education, makes demands on children which often produce some evidence of stress. At present the proportion of children with breakdown from stress sufficiently disturbing to parents and teachers to cause them to seek medical advice is small. A physical handicap, chronic or episodic illness, a specific learning disability, a poor socio-economic environment or deprivation of 'normal' family life, any or all of these make the child especially vulnerable. Health and education suffer and the result may be anti-social behaviour and delinquency. The influence of school absence and of variation in the effectiveness of educational methods in different kinds of school has always to be remembered in considering survey results. So, too, does the difficulty of deciding when a child's behaviour is 'deviant'.

The NCB survey did not reveal so definite a correlation between physical disorder and either behaviour and adjustment or educational attainment as in the Isle of Wight. The survey used the Bristol Social Adjustment Guide to group children as 'stable', 'unsettled' and 'maladjusted'. This depends on the summation of a number of scores and these in turn depend on the teacher's assessment. The investigation concentrated on the extreme 6 per cent of children with the highest ('worst') scores. In 1971 this would have included about 50 000 seven-year-old children. The syndrome of unforthcomingness, depression, withdrawal, anxiety or hostility towards adults or children, unconcern, restlessness or emotional tension, provide unusual reasons for medical consultation. On the other hand, the elements in deviant behaviour used in the Isle of Wight survey possess a more medical flavour. Parents do seek medical advice when their children fidget, truant, steal, bite their nails, suck their thumbs, stutter, and even more readily when they do not eat or sleep, have 'stomach-ache', bilious attacks and wet or soil themselves. All of these are common symptoms and all doctors should know how to assess their importance in relation to health, emotional adjustment and educational success as well as in relation to family psycho-pathology.

The needs of children with emotional and psychiatric disorders demand more than can be provided by a Health Service or the doctors working in it. Although in prevention, health education, mothercraft and fathercraft, infant care and the management of the pre-school child are all concerned, housing, employment, educational and social policies are also implicated. While further research is necessary, much of what is already known has failed to reach the population at large in which are included doctors, nurses and health visitors. A great deal depends on the economic health of the community, on legislation by central government and on the extent to which local authorities are willing and able to carry out what is centrally recommended. Finally, success and failure are determined by the attitudes, the skills and the conscientiousness of the 'workers in the field', and their numbers. The priority is to define objectives. Thereafter it may become possible to penetrate barriers created by traditional attitudes and cultural habits. Meanwhile much can be done to help that part of the vulnerable child population which is already under medical treatment or surveillance by recognizing their vulnerability.

Much is done for those children and families where recognizable psychiatric syndromes require treatment by psychiatrists. Howells estimates that 'psychosis accounts for less than one per cent of patients seen at child psychiatric clinics'. This leaves a vast acreage of emotional problems at present largely untilled.

The content of psychiatric work for children and their families may be described in three categories:

1. Psychiatric disorders of children and adolescents including not only psychoses, but also neurotic, conduct and anti-social disorders as categorized by Rutter (*v. sup.*).
2. Mental handicap and severe mental handicap including preliminary diagnosis, full assessment and continuing management both within the community and with custodial care of some kind (see Chapter 13).
3. The psychiatric or emotional reactions which affect children and their families, and which sometimes form the primary cause of disease, accident and handicap. More frequently they appear as secondary complications. It is this category that is of the most importance for the paediatrician and for the general practitioner.

The size of the problem is formidable. The time and the staff needed for assessment is great and treatment sessions involving the child and his family cannot be hurried. The questions arise—who is to do the work and where should the work be done? The Danish figures quoted by Howells suggest that each year at least 30 000 children in England and Wales have serious psychiatric problems. The Isle of Wight figures indicate more than 100 000 10- and 11-year-olds with psychiatric problems of whom over 10 000 need specialized psychiatric treatment. It is difficult to see how the problem of numbers can be solved without the reintegration of psychological medicine into the rest of medicine. If paediatrics is truly concerned with the health of the child in the context of his family and with the child's realization of his full potential, child psychiatry must be an integral part of paediatrics, the child psychiatrist must be a kind of paediatrician, and paediatricians, whether consciously or sub-consciously, cannot avoid involvement in the practice of some parts of phycho-paediatrics, especially those described in paragraphs 2 and 3 above. When paediatricians take responsibility, as they are bound to do, for children with acute nephritis or with congenital heart disease, they seek at times the help of some who have explored more deeply or who are attempting research in nephrology and cardiology. The relationship between the general paediatrician and the paediatric psychiatrist need differ in no way from his relationship with the paediatric nephrologist or cardiologist.

The general practitioner has his accustomed part to play as the doctor of first contact. It is for him to separate from the temporary and often mono-symptomatic behaviour problems and functional disturbances the child and the family who need more of his time than can be spared out of a busy surgery. From this selected group he will need to refer some to the paediatrician and some to the child psychiatrist. He should be familiar with family interactions and he should be conscious of the emotional element contained in every consultation, even in a routine examination. His training and experience should enable him to play his part in treating many of these problems.

The third of the above categories of psychiatric work remains an area in much of which neither paediatricians nor child psychiatrists have accepted primary responsibility and which has only recently been seriously explored. There are especially the many situations which, although arising from conditions essentially paediatric in the classical sense, contain strong emotional or psychological elements. Among these are the following:

1 Those connected with the birth of dead, abnormal or handicapped babies.
2 Repeated trauma whether accidental or non-accidental.
3 Deprivation syndromes causing physical, emotional and intellectual stunting.
4 Reactions to episodic and chronic disorders and their long term care, for example:
   (a) Asthma, epilepsy, cystic fibrosis of the pancreas, haemophilia;
   (b) Severe anatomical defects such as those associated with myelomeningocele, absence or deformity of limbs, muscular dystrophy and other crippling conditions.
5 Those connected with the birth of babies to unmarried mothers and with adoption.
6 Those where parental psychopathology and mental illness affect the care of children and the future of the family.
7 Those connected with communication and learning difficulties.
8 Those connected with genetically determined diseases, and the emotional effects of amniocentesis, of predictive fetal diagnosis and of the request for abortion.

The treatment of the child and of his family must remain in the hands of one person, but for assessment and for the prescribing of therapeutic policy a team is essential. Skill in developmental assessment and in identifying specific disabilities which can handicap learning is basic. There exists an unfortunate and hampering disagreement about the ideal function for the various professionals whose work overlaps in this clinical/educational area. Clarification of roles between psychiatrists, neurologists, social workers, psychologists and paediatricians is overdue. Here again defining objectives comes first and when the nature and extent of the task has been estimated, a decision should be possible about who does what. The development of intellect, the perceptual and motor skills, the presence of sickness and neurological deficits, family making skills, socio-economic circumstances and school life, are so interwoven that the basic problem or problems cannot always or easily be identified. At least the parents and the school teachers should be made aware of what is involved.

Within the total population of children with emotional and psychiatric problems who do require help, a few syndromes can be recognized and quantified.

Autistic behaviour. Lotter (1966) studied the 8- to 10-year-old population of the old County of Middlesex by questionnaire and case record, and by interview with selected children and informants. He based his diagnosis on the child's failure to respond to people in a normal way, the presence of repetitive-ritualistic behaviour and abnormal movements, and failure of speech and communication. He found mental illness in many families and both a higher social class bias and educational and intellectual superiority in the mother in all social classes. His suggested prevalence of children displaying autistic behaviour is 4.5 per 10 000, of whom two thirds were judged to have a severe mental handicap (IQ below 55). In 1971 there should have been some 360 affected children entering the school population. About 5250 children would at some time during childhood have had autistic symptoms of sufficient severity to be clinically diagnosed, 3500 of school and 1750 of pre-school age. All would have suffered language retardation. In 1970, 700 were in hospitals for the mentally subnormal (House of Lords Debate, 1970).

Cerebral palsy. Among the school population in 1971 this would have affected 19 400 children (2.5 per 1000) of whom 7750 (1 per 1000) would have been severely mentally handicapped. Among 5-year-old school entrants, the corresponding numbers would have been 2000 and 800.

Severe language retardation. This is found in less than 1 per 1000

(Edinburgh, Ingram's figure is 0.71 per 1000; Isle of Wight, Rutter's figure is 0.8 per 1000). About 5 per cent of children at school entry have unintelligible speech and 1 per cent have serious language retardation (for 1971 40 000 and 8000 respectively at 5 years).

In all of these groups, as well as for those enumerated in Chapter 13 under Mental Handicap, much individual and family emotional strain and disturbance are inevitable.

One outcome as well as promoter of family stress is *non-accidental trauma* (see p. 229), American estimates of prevalence give 300 to 400 children affected per million of population. An approximate estimate for the 1971 total populations lies between 12 000 and 15 000. Much remains concealed within accidents and especially repeated accidents and unexpected death in the first three years of life. Abuse should be more widely suspected. Jackson (1972) working in a hospital well alerted to this possibility found on a retrospective study of 100 cases of physical injury under the age of 12 years that the diagnosis had been overlooked in 18, all under the age of 2 years. Excessive crying, anorexia, frequent smelly stools, failure to gain weight in the early months of life are often warning evidence and it is to be hoped that the behaviour of mothers towards feeding and handling their babies in the newborn period will provide clues so that preventive action may be taken. This requires further study which should involve midwives and the obstetric nursing staff.

Defects of *fine manipulation,* important in handicapping learning and associated with poor motor control or spatial appreciation, cannot yet be quantified. Nor is it yet possible to predict the children whose failure easily to learn to read will lead through frustration to severe emotional stress and even refusal to accept education. The direction of surveillance and assessments towards these practical ends will lead to earlier diagnosis, to some possibility of quantification and to prevention of the secondary ill effects.

'Child Guidance Service'

According to theories generally accepted today, disturbed behaviour has strong psychological determinants. When the effect is mainly within the family, medical advice is likely to be sought. When either the smooth course of education is interrupted or school behaviour becomes undisciplined, the local authority educational or medical service takes responsibility. When anti-social behaviour reaches out into the community, the police and the courts are often involved. The resulting symptoms of breakdown do not necessarily reflect either the basic faults and stresses or determine the scene of the problem, whether home, school or community. The logical solution would be to have for all the disturbances of behaviour or learning one assessment and therapy service, which contains physicians, psychotherapists, psychologists and social workers with easy access to other medical, pedagogic, social and legal specialists. Historical piecemeal development has led to a variety of clinics, some of which are attached to hospitals, but most of which relate to the education authority. The development of medical interest in these problems and a chronic shortage of skilled manpower might make a long-term aim the unification of these psychological services. The logical place would then be association with the National Health Service Departments of Child Health.

The Summerfield Report (1968), dealing with psychologists in education services, has concurred in stating that 'The psychological needs of children at school and *in their families* should continue to be the focus of psychological work in the education service'. The Report goes on to suggest a need for more of their work to be done both during the pre-school years and also for a year or two after school has been left. When to these are added work for the Court in co-operation with the probation officers and in training centres for the mentally handicapped, that part of the problem that concerns school education is seen in a new perspective within a much larger picture.

The need for radical re-thinking of techniques and places gains support from the figures and estimates in Table 12.1, which demonstrate both high demand for and low supply of personnel in the education services alone.

Table 12.1. Child psychological services education authority personnel, proposed and actual (Summerfield 1968)

	Underwood 1965	1966	1969	*Project* 1971	1975
	Proposed per				
School children in thousands	45	7092.2	7387.8	7756.6	9088.4
Psychiatrists	1	158 (110)	164 (108)	175	202
Educational psychologists	2	315 (324)	328 (279)	349	404
Psychiatric social workers	3	473 (160)	492	524	606
E.P.'s at 1 per 10 000 (Summerfield)	4.5	709	738	776	909

Note: In brackets are actual staff in full-time equivalents.

CHAPTER 13

Mental handicap

For the assessment of the health needs of mentally handicapped children a separation is necessary into two essentially different groups, mild handicap and severe. The latter group includes moderate, severe and profound mental retardation in USA and WHO terminology. The separation is bound in practice to be somewhat artificial, but it does make possible some estimate of prevalence and of the quantity and the quality of the care required. To a material extent, the separation depends on the now suspect results of intelligence testing. The IQ, it is generally agreed, is not a fixed index but is capable of both improvement and deterioration during childhood. Broadly, the mildly handicapped are in the IQ area of 50–70, while the severely handicapped are below 50. Expressed in another way, the mildly handicapped extend from 2 to 3 standard deviations below the mean of 100, the severe beyond 3 SD. The separation gains further justification, because most of the mild group are physically normal, in contrast with the severe group, in whom pathological lesions of the brain are commonly found, although their basis is not always known.

Social, economic and emotional factors certainly play their part in determining the health need, and so do the presence, the nature and the severity of any physical handicap.

MILD MENTAL HANDICAP

Mild mental handicap, as Kushlick (1968) has observed, 'is a temporary incapacity related largely to educational difficulties experienced in school'. As the distribution of intelligence measured by IQ in a normal child population follows a Gaussian curve, some 2 per cent would be expected to fall into the mildly handicapped group. In 1971 this would have amounted to a little less than 148 000 in the total school population (5–14 years). The actual numbers are unknown, since only those requiring supervision or recognized as needing special education are identified. Their health needs for all forms of medical care should not differ materially from those of the remaining 98 per cent of school children. Complications arising from family emotional stress and any consequent behaviour disorders could be reduced if education for success replaced education for failure in schools with a careful search for and encouragement of attainments of which the child is capable and with the adoption of special teaching methods.

Developmental surveillance of large populations will reveal to what extent delays in achievement in infancy are related to mild mental handicap and the reliability of infant assessments as predictors of educational difficulties. The identification of such babies is likely to add to parental anxieties and would be cruel and harmful unless linked with parent counselling and detailed instruction in the best methods of developing such intellectual potential as the baby possesses.

In the preventive programme the needs of the mildly handicapped appear to be social and cultural rather than medical. Some evidence exists for a genetic factor but stronger epidemiological evidence favours cultural deprivation. Clinically normal children with IQ 50–70 are virtually absent from the higher social classes and come largely from Classes IV and V. Insufficient language stimulation in infancy and early childhood may be a factor, creating sometimes a gap that cannot later be filled. So, too, may be the kind of 'minimal cerebral dysfunction' associated with the disadvantaged ante- and peri-natal care of these two classes.

Most of the children in the mild group are later able to live adult lives that are socially and economically independent, to marry, to found stable families and to become successful citizens. Their contribution to failure in marriage, to broken homes and to such social problems as illegitimacy and child abuse is unascertained. Whatever the size of this contribution, the possession of limited intelligence is at present regarded as less likely to cause difficult or delinquent behaviour in adolescent or adult life than a childhood spent, deprived of love, in a disrupted family or in an inadequately staffed institution.

The general practitioner is likely to meet with mental handicap so seldom in his practice that he cannot be expected to develop expertise. He will become concerned about the infants whose surveillance reveals delayed development. He should be able to recognize or at least be suspicious about babies and children who show the peculiar physical characteristics of microcephaly, mongolism, cretinism and cerebral palsy. He must in these ways play an invaluable part in case finding. There must also be a place for the paediatrically orientated general practitioner in the multi-discipline assessment and supervision units. Probably his most valuable, and it may be a unique, function is to gain access to and achieve the confidence of those families in his practice whose reaction to the presence of a mentally handicapped child is to isolate themselves from the community in a way that is detrimental to the mental health of the whole family.

Local health authority doctors and doctors in the school health service have a statutory duty to perform in the assessment, placement and the continuing management of mentally handicapped children. The discharge of this duty requires hospital assessment centres backed up by visits to the homes and families from skilled workers in the community child health and school health services. Care based on the home becomes more easily bearable as well as more effective when parents are given training in the best ways of handling their mentally handicapped children and when some respite is afforded through day care in day nurseries, special units and special classes in school.

The role of the paediatrician

All practising paediatricians must be involved in the diagnosis, the case-finding, the assessment and the surveillance of mentally handicapped children, both mild and severe. They should possess both experience and expertise in 'telling the parents' and in helping families to adjust to the emotional strains of the early months. What else they can do remains open for discussion. Paediatric neurologists and paediatric psychiatrists together with paediatricians with a vocation towards psycho-paediatrics will insist on playing their valuable and continuing pastoral part, but even if all paediatricians in all grades were prepared to lead teams, the case load alone would defeat the enterprise.

If a *chronic handicap annexe* were attached, as suggested by the BPA, to every main paediatric hospital or department, the in-patient study and assessment of mentally handicapped children could be carried out there under paediatric supervision. Some paediatricians lack vocation for this work, but others could be encouraged to make it a speciality. Such specialists could achieve much in improving the lot of their patients, by organizing the assessment teams, linking with social working agencies, advising the proposed new residential hostels and perhaps taking charge of some of the remaining 'mental subnormality' hospitals. As teachers they could play an important part in under- and post-graduate education and they could supervise and encourage much needed epidemiological and therapeutic research in conjunction with university departments of community medicine, pharmacology and psychology.

Other trained staff, whose responsibilities are as great as those of the medically qualified, include clinical educational psychologists, specialized 'remedial' teachers, physiotherapists, speech therapists, play therapists, as well as laboratory workers. Occupational therapy has an important part to play if directed to the development of personality, social adjustment and preparation for life in whatever environment will be appropriate for the child. The paediatrician practising psycho-paediatrics would contribute also to the education of these workers.

The ultimate objectives

The aim implicit in this chapter is to secure for the mentally handicapped and for his family as much peace of mind, as much educational progress and as much physical care as is possible. Early diagnosis, counselling, surveillance, training, specialized medical and educational services appear as the basic necessities in order to assist the child and his family to live at peace emotionally within society. Such helps are unavailable to many and even were they provided they would fall far short of achieving ultimate objectives. These are four. First, a positive one, comes the development to his full potential and to the maximum independence of every handicapped child by the use of specialized educational techniques in which the close co-operation of parents forms a vital element. Second, a negative one, comes the avoidance of preventable disabilities, physical and emotional, that result from primary handicaps through faulty attitudes of mind and faulty techniques of training and management. Third, is the unresolved problem of lowering the incidence of mental handicap by optimal obstetric care and a combination of family planning and abortion, making use of amniocentesis. Fourth, comes wide-ranging research.

If the figures are accepted that at any one time there are 150 000 mildly and 50 000 severely mentally handicapped children aged 0–14 years, making a total of 200 000 individuals and their families, the question arises whether the medical care of so large a group does not justify the establishment of a new speciality.

The work of the general practitioner is the provision of primary care. Perhaps by developmental surveillance he will contribute to the identification of babies liable to later educational handicaps, but this work will remain chiefly in the hands of the community orientated doctor. The paediatrician has the same tasks with the additional responsibility for neonatal care. At present it is often left to him to advise on methods of encouraging the development of intellectual potential. Neither he nor the general practitioner may be the appropriate person to perform this task, which needs the skill of the expert psychologist, the teacher and the school doctor. Health education to encourage improved ante-natal attendance by the expectant mother and obstetric organization to extend the highest standard of obstetric management to the lower socio-economic groups also seem relevant.

SEVERE MENTAL HANDICAP

Severe mental handicap arises sometimes from an identifiable aetiological agent, but it is not always recognizable at birth and its occurrence remains often unpredictable and unavoidable. Known factors include chromosomal abnormalities, fetal infection and inborn errors of metabolism. A small steady contribution is made by neonatal and infant bacterial meningitis, some forms of encephalitis, thyroid deficiency, intracranial haemorrhage, either from true accident or child abuse, lead poisioning and incomplete resuscitation after anaesthetic 'death' or 'death' from physical agents.

Accurate diagnosis is made extremely difficult in the presence of neurological deficits handicapping movement and of disorders of communication and language, severe auditory or visual defects and profound emotional and behavioural disturbance.

Apart from the frequency of pathological lesions in the central nervous system, severe mental handicap differs from mild by its even distribution among the social classes and its positive association, not necessarily a causative one, with low birth weight.

Table 13.1. Places for children aged 0–15 years
(From Better services for the mentally handicapped, HMSO 1971)

Type of service	*Required per 100 000 total population*	*Total*	*Provided total*
Day care or education for children under 5 years	8	3 900	500 (estimated)
Education for school age children:			
In community:			
(i) living in the community	56	27 400	
(ii) coming from hospital	6		23 400 (i, ii and 2 900 bracketed)
In hospital:		2 900	
(iii) for in-patients	7	3 400	4 600
(iv) for day patients	6	2 900	200 (estimated)
Residential care in the community (including short stay):			
(i) in residential homes (LA and private)	10	4 900	1 800
(ii) in foster-homes etc.	2	1 000	100
Hospital treatment:			
(i) for in-patients	13	6 400	7 400 (allotted in NHS)
(ii) for day patients	6	2 900	200 (estimated)

Table 13.2. Staff of hospitals and hospital units for the mentally handicapped, September 1969
(From Better services for the mentally handicapped, p. 23)

Whole time equivalents		*Average ratio of staff to patients*	*Range of ratios (hospitals of 300 beds or more)*	
			Highest	*Lowest*
All medical staff	321	1:192	1:72	1:400
Nurses:				
qualified	8 754	1:3.86	1:2	1:6.2
other	6 475			

Table 13.3. Professional staff available in England and Wales from which must come the care of the mentally handicapped in a total population of 100 000 (Kushlick 1972)

GP	40
LHAMO	5
Paediatricians or child psychiatrists	1
Physicians	1.8
Psychiatrists	1.5
Educational psychologists	1
Social workers	12+
Home helps	63+
Health visitors	12+
Home nurses	18+
Teachers	5+

Prevalence of severe mental handicap

In 'Better Services for the Mentally Handicapped' (Cmmd. 4683,HMSO 1971) the number of the severely mentally handicapped in the 0–14-year-old population in England and Wales is estimated to be 50 000 (100 per 100 000 total population). Planning figures for these children according to the expected type of service required are listed in Table 13.1–13.3

1 The majority of the severely mentally handicapped have become known to the social agencies by the age of 15 years.
2 The prevalence in the age group 15 to 19 is found to be 4 per 1000 population; because of the reduced survival rate at each age, the prevalence for the total population is likely to be between 2 and 3 per 1000. The estimated rate for children under 15 is 4 per 1000.

3 Surveys have shown that at present only about 5 per cent of children assessed as severely mentally handicapped can achieve social and economic independence in adult life (Tizard 1958); the majority remain dependent.

4 Dependence by itself does not indicate the need for hospital care. McKeown and Teruel (1970) assessed the feasibility of discharging patients from Birmingham hospitals for the mentally subnormal. They found that 1 in 7 did not in fact require hospital care. Yet for the majority, home was unavailable on account of poor social conditions, illness of the mother or because the family was unwilling or unable to take the responsibility. The case for custodial care in hostel type accommodation is unanswerable.

5 Mongol children (birth incidence 1.5 per 1000) account for one quarter to one third of the severely mentally handicapped. Some 10 per cent achieve an IQ above 50 and these, together with the mongol mosaics who may reach 70 or higher, can be grouped with the mildly mentally handicapped for education and care.

Cerebral palsy is said to affect 2 per 1000 of all children, a population of 23 350 in 1971 (0–14 years: total 11 676 000). One half or 11 600 would have had an IQ of below 70 and one quarter or 5800 below 50. The incidence, the prevalence and the health needs of children with seizures, must be borne in mind in any discussion of the mentally handicapped, but with present knowledge quantification is beyond reach. The prevalence of children with epilepsy is shown elsewhere (see p. 155).

Surveys in Wessex, Newcastle and Camberwell give some indication of the amount of physical care and supervision required (Table 13.4).

The number of severely mentally handicapped children living at home who have physical handicaps or behaviour difficulties is less than the numbers of those who are away from home. Yet a substantially greater proportion remain severely incontinent and need assistance over personal living. Perhaps parental over-solicitude hinders the handicapped child's efforts at independence or perhaps skill in training techniques is lacking. Whichever is the correct interpretation, these findings suggest that much more could and should be done to instruct parents and to help them with the day to day care of their mentally handicapped children.

A working party of the Paediatric Society of the South East Metropolitan Region published in 1962 a paper on the needs of mentally handicapped children, which have much in common with the needs of children with physical handicaps. In both groups paediatricians and general practitioners have parts to play as members of multi-disciplinary

Table 13.4. The need for physical care and supervision
(expressed as rates per 100 000 total population aged 0–14 years)
This Table from 'Better services for the mentally handicapped' is based on surveys in Wessex, Newcastle and Camberwell.

Place of residence	*Degree of mental handicap*	*Non-ambulant*	*Behaviour difficulties requiring constant supervision*	*Severely incon-tinent*	*Needing assistance to feed, wash and other*	*No physical handicap or severe behaviour difficulties*	*Incapacity not assessed*	*Total*
Home	Severe	10.49	4.83	5.00	15.90	12.79	0.73	49.74
Hospital or other residential care	Severe	6.10	4.86	3.65	3.63	1.69	0.10	20.03
	Mild	0.34	0.88	0.15	0.23	3.85	0.21	5.55
Total		16.81 (16.93)	10.27 (10.57)	8.75 (8.80)	19.68 (19.76)	17.04 (18.33)	1.04	72.90 (75.32)

teams. A BPA working party has also produced a report, and the following list of needs, based on these two reports, lends some support to Tizard's view that in supplying the needs of the mentally handicapped, 'Paediatricians could assume a leading role in what is properly their province.' Their role is less easy to define in achieving the BPA's expressed visionary goal—'To eradicate mental handicap in childhood'. A more realistic aim would be to reduce to the smallest degree the unhappiness, the tensions and the wastage of potential produced by the presence in a family of a mentally handicapped child.

THE CARING NEEDS OF MENTALLY HANDICAPPED CHILDREN AND THEIR FAMILIES

The parents must try to provide the security of a stable family life with the approximate mixtures of love and discipline, and of protection, help and stimulation towards independence.

The dangers to be avoided are rejection on one hand and over-solicitude on the other, isolation of the family unit, and both physical and mental fatigue.

Apart from sustaining morale, their counsellor should instruct them in the training techniques aimed at developing independent living. Additional needs may be for home help, suitable housing, and finance, and arrangements for short-term residential care to relieve parents and siblings. Educational help is needed for placement in a school suitable to the child's intellectual potential and his physical competence.

Psychiatric help may be needed for an acceptance of and adjustment to the child's handicap.

The child needs, besides more or less provision of what is detailed above, medical help in primary care for acute illness and accident. Further medical and special therapeutic help is needed for any additional motor or sensory handicaps, such as cerebral palsy, defects of sight and hearing and other perceptual learning deficits, for epilepsy, for incontinence and for behaviour disorders. The latter may require preventive psychiatric help.

Provision is required for total preliminary and for continuing assessment, for day care in a nursery or special centre, and for residential care in a hospital, with short stay for assessment or long stay for medical or complex nursing and therapeutic care.

Follow-on care and assessment are needed aimed at placement in adolescent and adult life with the appropriate amount of protection and the appropriate type of employment.

Provision required to fulfil these needs

Diagnosis:

(a) Preliminary diagnosis of mental handicap follows neonatal assessment or developmental delay noted in a surveillance clinic or leading to a 'delay' consultation.

(b) Full assessment to discover all associated defects, such as neuromuscular (cerebral palsy), epilepsy, visual and auditory, perceptual learning, metabolic or chromosomal.

Surveillance:

(c) Definition of a programme for supervision, periodic (annual) reassessment, appropriate education and preparation for independent life: genetic counselling: parental morale support: special therapy.

Day centre or hostel:

(d) For general care, for advice and discussion, for habilitation, physio-, occupational or speech therapy, medical treatment.

Hospital:

(e) For primary care, acute illness or accident, for short-stay assessment, for long-stay care.

Employment centre:

(f) For special placement for the mentally handicapped.

Research:

(g) All aetiological aspects from epidemiological to biochemical and chromosomal, and into therapeutic and educational techniques.

General management of the severely mentally handicapped

Suspicion of severe mental handicap will arise in many babies and infants during either the neonatal period or later periodic surveillance. Day to day needs will be met in the first instance by the paediatrician or the general practitioner who originally identifies the handicap. At some point in time a fuller assessment will be undertaken in the local assessment centre or in the local paediatric out-patient department. Sometimes a more complex assessment in the regional assessment centre will be needed. The detection of motor and sensory handicaps in addition to the mental handicap has an essential place.

Support for the parents in accepting and adjusting to the diagnosis, of the utmost importance, and in management and training of the child, will be given not only by the doctor making the diagnoses, but also by the health visitor or other social worker, provided by statutory service or by voluntary society. The help of the geneticist may also be needed.

Community services for the training, education and recreation of the handicapped child are the responsibility of the local authority services. The health department will supervise an efficient follow-up, although this is rendered difficult by the high rate of population movement especially in urban areas.

CHAPTER 14

Cerebral palsy and epilepsy

CEREBRAL PALSY

For the attempt to quantify cerebral palsy and to identify its demands on health care, Rutter's definition (1970) has been adopted—that it is 'an unequivocally pathological motor disorder in which there was evidence of a non-progressive lesion above the brain stem'. This definition applies to the clinical results of the disorder on the immature brain and does not exclude the sensory, psychological and educational elements, which sometimes are more disabling than those motor elements which mark with their signature the affected child.

The lesion, which is usually present at birth, is regarded as congenital, although it may be acquired from fetal disease. The diagnosis may not be made within the first eighteen months of life. Every reported series includes a few whose disorder, acquired later, followed one of a group of diseases, some of which are preventable and for all of which treatment is capable of improvement. Prevalence rates, therefore, vary in different age groups.

An early American figure of incidence in the days when serious medical attention was beginning to be focused on these previously neglected children was as high as 5.9 per thousand births (Schenectady Study 1949). In the same period in Birmingham, Asher and Schonell (1950) gave a prevalence of only 1 per thousand school children. Out of 466 suspected children, they had accepted the diagnosis in 400. They listed 51 of the 400 (13 per cent) as acquired and of these 38 per cent (19) followed kernicterus, 4.75 per cent of the whole group. Infantile meningitis caused eleven, all severely mentally handicapped. Since 1950 kernicterus has diminished, obstetric care has improved and the science of neonatology has found practical applications in the care of the newborn. Grace Woods' reporting (1963) of a lowered incidence in Bristol is hardly surprising with a decrease from 2.5 per 1000 live births in 1948–1953 down to 0.9 in 1958–1962. The failure of Griffiths and Barrett (1967) to find any decline in Birmingham is no reason for pessimism since their comparison was between children born in 1950–54 with those born 1955–59. Their mean incidence figure for the later period was 1.3 per 1000 live births. The National Child Development Study reported 2.5 per 1000 total births in the cohort born in 1958 with a 7-year-old prevalence of 2.3 per 1000. For the present calculation the Isle of Wight figure for prevalence in the school population in 1965 has been adopted, 2.9 per 1000, 2.6 congenital and 0.3 acquired. To risk exaggerating the size of the problem is to err on the side of wisdom. On the other hand reports in the literature suggest that this figure is too high and is certainly now capable of a considerable reduction.

The success of neonatologists in their struggle to defeat the ill effects of hypoxia and hypoglycaemia must surely reduce the perinatal incidence unless current ideas about the aetiology of brain damage are wrong or unless increased knowledge and improved practice fail to spread within the health service. A corresponding decline in prevalence is expected to follow the decline in incidence as the new and more safely managed cohorts of newborns enter the child population.

In the acquired group a combination of the prevention of iso-immunization in rhesus negative women with availability of proper paediatric and laboratory skills for all newborn babies at risk of jaundice should virtually eliminate kernicterus. Neonatal meningitis, not always easy to recognize in its early stages, and sometimes, as with group B streptococci, having a devastating effect on the brain, present a much more difficult problem. The successful management of sub-dural haematoma and the prevention of serious child abuse make their contribution. Acute infantile hemiplegia remains, like neonatal meningitis, a problem for further research.

To know incidence and prevalence is not enough. The problems of parent counselling and of supporting advice arise in all the families. The other needs vary from handling a completely bedfast 'spastic' and severely mentally handicapped child, helpless and with no prospect of education or of an independent future to securing for a moderately disabled child, with hemiplegia and an average intelligence, the opportunity for a sound education leading to appropriate employment. The Isle of Wight figure of 35 affected children does not provide a good basis for subdivision into neurological types nor of associated sensory defects. Nor can conclusions rest on the 36 alive at 7 years in the National Child Development Study 1958 Cohort.

Unfortunately, no good studies exist of children in England and Wales large enough for the purpose of quantifying health needs. Guidance must be sought elsewhere. Table 14.1 relates the two Scottish reports of Henderson (1961) and of Ingram (1964) with Hansen's (1960) most practical study from Denmark. Henderson took 240 cases between 0 and 21 years in Dundee and the eastern region of Scotland (born between 1939 and 1961). He gives a prevalence rate for 5 to 14 years of 2.04 per 1000,

Table 14.1. Cerebral palsy

		Hansen 1960 N=2621	*Henderson* 1961 N=240	*Ingram* 1954–64 1964 N=200	*NCB* 1972 N=36	*Calculated populations* 1971 N=22 500
	Birth years	1925–53	1939–61	1938–52	1958	1954–64
	Birth incidence	1.3/1000	(0–14) 1.8/1000	—	2.5/1000 total	—
	Prevalence (years)	85.6	(5–14) 2.04/1000	(5–14) 2.5/1000	(7) 2.3/000	(5–14) 2.9/1000
Type	Spastic		78.3	83.0		19 250
			Mixed, mainly spastic 9.5			
	Athetoid	9.3 } 13.3	7.5 } 9.6	dyskinesia		} 3 000
	Ataxia and tremor	4.0 }	2.1 }	10.0		}
	Unspecified	1.1	2.6	7.0		
Motor handicap	Slight	41.0	42.7	52.5		9 250
	Moderate	40.9	34.8	33.5		9 200
	Severe	18.10	22.5	14.0		4 050
Intelligence	Normal (above 70 IQ)	47.7 (N=223)	51.6	55.0	52.8	11 800
	Retarded (50–69 IQ)	20.4	22.9	24.0	36.1	8 200
	Severely subnormal (below 50 IQ)	27.1	22.3	21.0	11.1	2 250
	Unclassified	4.8	3.9	—	—	—
Defect	Epilepsy	22.2	25.0	31.6	—	5 000
	Speech	41.7	27.0	52.9	—	10 000
	Hearing	4.0 (N=70)	23.0	—	—	—
	Oculo-motor	21.2	—	—	—	4 500
	Ophthalmological	—	58.4	—	—	13 000

and he points out that many were not diagnosed for the first 18 months of life. 28 acquired cases (12.1 per cent) included kernicterus (7), meningitis (7) and acute infantile hemiplegia (7). As with selection of cases in many other reported series, a large number of children (in Edinburgh 20 per cent of the total of 301) were wrongly suspected of having cerebral palsy. Presumably these represent other forms of neurological deficit.

Ingram (1964) reported ascertainment of 144 patients in Edinburgh born between 1938 and 1948 and studied in 1952–53. He based his report on 200 traced survivors among the Edinburgh patients and 75 from the series in Dundee and its environs. He adopted a prevalence rate of 2.5 patients per 1000 of population aged 5 to 14 years. Hansen (1960) based his report on cerebral palsy in Denmark on the study of a population aged 2 to 30 years, born between 1925 and 1953, with a birth incidence of 1.3 per 1000 live births. Applying the results of his analysis, the more precise health needs of the affected population can be identified and measured.

Table 14.1, while illustrating differences possibly depending on variations in method, is consistent enough to allow some applications to the 1971 population. Something of the order of 1000 babies should have been diagnosable within the early months of life and a further 350 would have needed careful and repeated examination because of suspicion of cerebral palsy. In the school population (5 to 14 years) Rutter's rate would have given about 22 500 diagnosed children of whom 9250 would have had only a slight physical handicap and 4000 a severe one, while about 800 would have been helpless (Hansen). Intelligence (NCB) would have been in the normal range for about half (11 800), retarded in about a third (8200) and severely subnormal in a tenth (2250). Between 5000 and 13 000 would have needed ophthalmological services, 5000 treatment and supervision for fits, and perhaps 10 000 speech therapy, although their ability to benefit would have depended on the level of intelligence. When the degree of improvement claimed by Woods in Bristol has spread to the whole population, the annual increment of diagnosed babies should drop to 800 and the number in the school population to less than half the present estimated 22 500, with a corresponding decrease in the other groups.

With regard to defects of hearing the difficulties of testing and the failure always to test both ears have probably prevented the full assessment of the size of the problem and, as expected, the numbers with known hearing defects increase when special attention is paid to diagnosis.

More subtle defects of both auditory and visual perception, which handicap the learning process are far from easy to identify in this group of children who have other neurological deficits. Expected progress in teaching techniques will increase the importance of the identification of these defects.

Health needs for cerebral palsied children

Prevention depends on availability and utilization of good antenatal and obstetric services, expert care of the newborn especially in the control of rhesus iso-immunization, hypoxia, hypoglycaemia and the management of the small-for-dates baby. What antenatal contribution could be made to the congenital cases by genetics and prediction remains to be discovered. Socio-economic factors do not seem to affect incidence, although they do affect progress.

A more effective identification of congenitally affected babies could be allied to preventive physiotherapy and exercises, using automatic postural responses in the first years of life to prevent the establishment of faulty postural reactions (Bobath 1966). Routine assessment and surveillance at special intervals for suspected patients should be part of the general plan. At some appropriate time a full assessment is necessary, involving intelligence, seeing, hearing, speech and a search for some other congenital defect.

During this early period, parents require morale support, instruction in the best methods of physically handling their babies and help to adjust to the facts of the situation. Depression, anxiety and guilt require explanation and treatment. The twin dangers of over-protection and rejection have to be consciously recognized and overcome, so that the maximum of self-care and independence is established both by day and by night. Much parental and family suffering is avoidable, both in relation to interaction between immediate members of the family and isolation from neighbours, friends and even close relatives. To achieve the right balance is essential for the mental health of the whole family. A greater provision of day care for the pre-school severely handicapped child would certainly help.

When the child reaches school age, school placement calls for complete assessment so that problems are recognized, understood and helped. Should there have been a failure of earlier full assessment, school entry provides a useful stimulus. In addition to the examinations for special deficits already mentioned, dental and orthopaedic attention may be required and seizures may need control by drugs.

The community has also a part to play. To spend time and trouble in school placement has long been accepted as a responsibility of the education authority. No less importance attaches to the home environment in which the handicapped child may safely develop his full potential. The ground floor, protected outside play space, suitable bathing and lavatory facilities provide the setting for the development of maximum independence, and sufficient space for the rest of the family relieves parents from the additional frustration and exhaustion that may make the bringing up of a severely handicapped child an unbearable burden.

As the child reaches adolescence he will need to have adjusted himself to his own handicaps and limitations and both to his difference from from the handicap-free child and to his resemblances so that he can accept himself and his situation. Career selection and training mark the end of the child health stage.

The activities of the general practitioner in families which contain children with cerebral palsy cannot be identified. His work when there is intercurrent disease would be classified under that disease heading. The ICD numbers 343 and 344, cerebral spastic infantile paralysis and other cerebral palsies, are unmentioned in the morbidity statistics (GPR). They feature among causes of death (57) in RGSR, and in HIPE the estimate is 1938. The Child Health Centre, the school clinic and the assessment centre are the places where most of the work is done with a good deal at periodic visits to the hospital out-patient department. When the general practitioner can help with advice over the problems of daily living and relieve anxieties about the child's future, he is performing an invaluable service which is difficult to record in statistical terms.

EPILEPSY

The definition of epilepsy varies between different surveys, but essentially there has to be evidence of Hughlings Jackson's 'sudden, violent, disorderly discharge of the brain cells'. The episode consists of impairment or loss of consciousness with or without convulsive movements or other abnormal behaviour. Grand mal, psychomotor (temporal lobe) and myoclonic epilepsy are all included, grand mal being by far the commonest. Between 80 and 90 per cent begin before the age of 20 years. The effectiveness of treatment, in its widest sense, during childhood and adolescence must, therefore, greatly influence the pattern of life which the patient will follow.

Acceptance into a survey demands at least one fit in a stated pre-survey period or the taking of regular anti-convulsant drugs. Convulsions are relatively common among children with severe mental handicap, cerebral palsy and other organic brain diseases, when general management is usually related to the basic handicap rather than to the convulsions.

Epilepsy is reputed to affect 4 out of every 1000 in the total population (Cohen Report 1956), sufferers amounting to between 195 000 and 200 000 in 1971. Livingston (1963) states that every individual may have a fit, and in fact about 5 per cent of all people do have a fit at some time of life (GP Survey 1960). Prevalence rates vary at different ages. Seizures, often repeated, occur in the first week of life and again as benign febrile convulsions during the second and third years. More serious are those that begin or recur around the time of puberty, the decade 15 to 24 years being a peak period of idiopathic epilepsy. At this time, many of the children who have or who have had petit mal produce grand mal seizures. For practical purposes, out of all those with seizures of one kind or another, the number of about 50 000 can be accepted for school children with epilepsy and without gross neurological disease. The Reid Committee (1969) adopted the figure of about 100 000 children of 16 years and under with 2 to 4 new cases per 1000 each year (1600 to 3200).

Among the Newcastle families 7.2 per cent of children had one or more fits during the first 5 years of life. Applied to 1971 this represents about 282 000, a large number that includes neonatal, symptomatic and febrile convulsions. Out of 61 affected children, 49 survived at 5 years, of whom 3 continued to have fits. If these small figures may be used, the expected number of children with epilepsy at 5 years out of the 282 000 who had had fits, would be 14 000. A survey of general practices reported in 1960 produced a prevalence rate at 5 to 14 years of 4.6 per 1000, some 35 000 in the school population. The Isle of Wight study accepted only those children who had had a definite fit since starting school, 8.9 per 1000 (69 030) and who, during the pre-survey year, had either had at least one fit (4.9/1000) or who had been on regular anti-convulsant drugs (4.0/1000). When all those with organic brain disease were excluded, the prevalence rate was 6.4 per 1000, yielding 49 642 among the 1971 school children. The NCB survey gives a 7-year-old prevalence of 6.2 per 1000, which means about 5000 entering the school population each year.

The aims of treatment are fivefold:

1 to reduce the number of seizures while avoiding the harmful effects of drugs,
2 to identify any neurological deficits or other disabilities and to take

appropriate steps to counter their effects,

3 to encourage the child to lead as full and normal a life at home and at school as his potential allows,

4 to encourage his acceptance on the basis of his capabilities by his family, his school and the community,

5 and to ensure that the child develops a balanced attitude towards himself and his disability.

The stage may be set by parental (and doctor's) attitudes towards infantile convulsions and these attitudes should be explored since they will set the pattern for the unpredictable few whose 'fits' continue into later childhood. Unwillingness to consult the doctor arises from fear of the label 'epileptic' and of the sanctions which are applied in school and in later life. The Newcastle observers expressed surprise that at the five-year follow-up one fifth of the parents of the children with fits had failed to seek medical advice. In the General Practice Survey (1960) less than one quarter of the children were referred to paediatricians for their fits, and these usually to obtain an electro-encephalogram.

The unpredictable loss of body control and impairment of consciousness, together with being labelled an 'epileptic' induces in the sufferer a feeling of being 'different'. Perceptual disorders, which impede learning, are relatively common. Gastaut (1965) found 'perceptive–motor' difficulties in one third of children with epilepsy studied, and Rutter *et al.* (1970) noted among 9- to 12-year-olds reading retardation of more than 28 months in 25 per cent compared with 4 per cent in the controls. Subclinical discharges, affecting attention if not impairing consciousness, may add to the strain imposed by education. When to these is added prohibition of a number of normal childhood activities, such as cycling, swimming and sport, and later car-driving, the growing person is under considerable emotional strain. Uncovenanted side-effects of anti-convulsant drugs may increase difficulties in adjustment, a matter of importance because emotional strain is itself a factor in precipitating convulsions. Prohibitions, like drugs, need careful prescription. Lennox has well said: 'Enemy epilepsy prefers to attack when the patient is off guard, sleeping, resting or idling.'

Since the synthesis of phenobarbitone half a century ago, doctors have accepted its value in suppressing convulsions, but have been preoccupied with finding better drugs. The attempt to suppress infrequent convulsions may not necessarily be to the patient's advantage, especially if anti-convulsant drugs cause behaviour disturbances or damp down learning ability. Indeed, Pryse-Phillips (1969) has suggested looking on convulsions as 'a kind of self-administered ECT'. Millichap (1968) has identified the indications for continuing drug treatment after febrile convulsions. Too much concentration on attempts to suppress further convulsions may lead to neglect of the other aims of treatment. The real objective is to bring up a child who is liable to recurrent fits to live a normal life and to receive education in readiness for doing a job and taking his place in the community.

Medical needs include careful selection of drugs for patients and of patients for drugs. Much wise counselling of parents and child, much explanation, encouragement and morale support are necessary and only such restriction of activities as is considered essential. Those who work mainly among people with epilepsy run the risk of being too bold by reason of their wish to 'normalize' the child's life, while those who lack experience or interest may err by forbidding as a matter of routine every activity which contains a possible danger.

The general practitioner should be responsible for routine supervision, which includes arranging for the regular taking of prescribed drugs, and the price he pays for the privilege is to take an active interest in the total management of the patient's problems. Referral to a centre for full assessment would be indicated to exclude an underlying disease, for children whose lives are disturbed by recurrent convulsions, and also when the family is disturbed and finds acceptance of the situation beyond its unaided powers. The Cohen Report recommended assessment in all cases at 4 years, so that the school medical officer could be notified although the label epileptic should not be used. It is no longer permissible to speak of epileptics: there are people with epilepsy or children with seizures.

The composition of the assessment team requires some further discussion. The Cohen Sub-Committee (1956) recommended that each regional hospital board should establish one diagnostic and treatment clinic for every million of the population and for each two million one long-term (over 3 months' stay) treatment and rehabilitation centre. This responsibility presumably belongs now to the area health authority. The clinic should be in the charge of a neurological physician and would need a paediatrician, a radiologist, a psychologist, full social services and electro-encephalography. There should be close contacts with the general practitioner and also with both the educational services and the youth employment officers. For assessment and for stabilization of drug treatment and for patients with severe behaviour problems including those with temporal lobe epilepsy, an in-patient unit of fifty beds could handle two hundred patients each year. The Reid Report (1969) has proposed five or six special centres for England and Wales. There has been no suggestion of separating children from adolescents or either from adults, but what is proposed is a separate epilepsy service.

Aggressive, anti-social or other 'bad' behaviour necessitates special school accommodation for some children with epilepsy. Separate from epileptic colonies, but linked with the special centres, these special schools would try to train the child with the aims of future employment and a return to home or hostel life. The existence of an unpleasant 'epileptic personality' is usually now regarded as a myth. Paediatric thinking would favour the view that parental anxiety and rejection combined with a child's feeling of insecurity and of being 'different' are likely to predispose to personality and behaviour problems, which to some extent and in theory are preventable.

The general reticence about epilepsy hinders sufferers from obtaining treatment in childhood and jobs in adolescence. There is, therefore, a place for further education of the public who should understand that the person with epilepsy properly treated can lead a normal life and engage in all but a few occupations. The treatment of the child should be aimed in this direction.

Epilepsy is 'a sufficiently major (*sic*) problem to demand that special medical provision be made for dealing with it' (Cohen Report 1956).

Health needs

Primary care for the original convulsion is usually provided by the general practitioner. Some circumstances in which the child will be already in contact with the paediatrician are when there has been neonatal illness, or when there is associated mental handicap or cerebral palsy. The convulsions may follow illness for which the child is in hospital, such as meningitis, encephalomyelitis or injury from accident or non-accidental trauma or may complicate Sturge-Weber syndrome, subacute sclerosing encephalitis or other degenerative brain diseases. The history, investigations or the passage of time will separate those children whose treatment has to be dominated by the occurrence of seizures.

Idiopathic epilepsy is first seen and treated by the general practitioner and he may call for help in excluding symptomatic epilepsy or when there are recurrences. The question of more or less routine immediate admission of infants following what are probably febrile convulsions needs study. The general practitioner uses his discretion in selecting patients for referral to the paediatrician or the paediatric neurologist. A short period of hospital attendance, as in- or out-patient, may be needed for assessment, for stabilization of anti-convulsive drugs and in the school years for psychometry, tests of psycho-linguistic ability, of fine manipulation and of specific perceptual learning disability. Such assessments should be available in the appropriate assessment centre.

The shock of disclosure of epilepsy to parents must always be remembered and the parents may even need psychotherapy to help them to adjust. Counselling may be necessary even when the child has infrequent seizures, since their unpredictable nature makes them difficult to live with. Genetic counselling may also be required.

Sooner or later the child returns to the general practitioner for supervision and for the supply of prescriptions which should be for small quantities. Dosage and effectiveness of anti-convulsant drugs need periodic review either by the general practitioner or at the hospital and one person must be responsible for the continuity of drug treatment and for seeking out the truant from appointments. The recent attention paid to phenobarbitone as an enzyme inducer may reveal hitherto unsuspected effects of its prolonged use.

Admission to school is an indication for assessment, if not previously conducted. The school medical officer, the educational welfare officer and the school teacher should be brought into the picture. At present only half the children with epilepsy are known to their teachers. Any prohibition of activities or special supervision should be agreed and the emotional stress of school entry and later of move from primary to secondary school should be lightened as much as possible. Holiday camp for the child may help the rest of the family.

During school years the child with epilepsy should have morale support and explanation, together with some early warning of inadvisable careers and limitations of normal activities. The school leaving interviews with doctor and youth employment officer are essential and assessment of suitability for a particular employment may be advisable in an industrial habilitation unit. In 1971, 9810 school children with epilepsy needed treatment or observation in England and Wales. In April 1972, 22 000 people with epilepsy were on the Disabled Persons' Register out of an estimated total of 91 000 in the working population.

Both Cohen (1956) and Reid (1969) Reports recommended special centres for epilepsy, Reid suggesting five or six supra-regional centres in England and Wales with the dual function of providing technical neurological and neurosurgical expertise and residential facilities for assessment, research and teaching. A multi-disciplinary team should be available at every district general hospital and in all hospitals with neurological and neurosurgical units. Personnel includes consultants, social workers, clinical psychologists, local authority staff and a disablement resettlement officer, and close contact should be maintained with general practitioners. There appears to be no reason why special teams and special centres for children should not be established at university department of paediatrics or child health. All that is written and said today stresses that the developing child is more important than his seizures.

Residential accommodation will be of two kinds, one for short-stay investigation and assessment and the second for longer stay when stabilization is difficult, life at home impossible or where anti-social and 'bad' behaviour make the child difficult to control. The aim should be rehabilitation towards discharge and, when home life is impossible or inadvisable, boarding out or hostel arrangements made. A need for some 'colonies' is likely to remain, but as far as possible, children with epilepsy should be integrated into the general handicapped group.

In 1971 there were 620 special school places for children with epilepsy and 680 children awaiting admission. About half of the children admitted remain for less than 2 years. Dunlop and Richmond studied 360 children in Lingfield in 1964 and found that 54 per cent had neurological dysfunction or damage (10 per cent a hemiplegia), 40 per cent were slow learners or were so clumsy as to make school work difficult, 25 per cent had speech defects, 11 per cent defects of vision and 4 per cent hearing loss. Psychological disturbances affected 64 per cent.

The general practitioner's work has been described. The 'average' practitioner with a 2500 list will have care of 18 to 20 people with epilepsy of whom more than half would be children. The Morbidity Survey gives rates of consultation per thousand population as 2.0 and 2.6 in the age groups 0–4 and 5–14, the actual numbers of consultation recorded between the 118 practitioners during the year being 167 (GPR). Although only a small proportion will present problems, he must appreciate their vulnerability. In a group practice some degree of specialization of responsibility for surveillance might be beneficial.

Health education remains of great importance. Not only should the patient and his immediate family understand the nature of epilepsy and the possibility of living a normal life with it, but the community, especially the school, must be similarly enlightened. The promise that a child with epilepsy can take a normal place in society cannot be fulfilled without the consent of society.

CHAPTER 15

Infectious diseases

Table 15.1 of notification of certain infectious diseases is taken from RGSR 1971 and includes those infections which were deemed preventable and were included at the time in the programme of routine immunization. Although measles vaccine was available and recommended during the second year of life, this infection greatly exceeded all the others. It should be observed that 5 per cent of the notified cases of measles occurred before the first birthday. The absence of small pox and the small

Table 15.1. Notification of certain infectious diseases (RGSR 1971, Table 30)

RGSR deaths			*Children under 15*
0	Typhoid fever	54	
0	Paratyphoid	32	
110	Acute meningitis	1 171	(236 under 1 year)
3	Scarlet fever	11 548	
26 (20 under 6 months)	Whooping cough	16 259	(9238 under 5 years, 56.8 per cent, 3733 under 2 years, and 976 or 6 per cent under 6 months; peak 2–4 years, 5505)
1	Diphtheria	10	
5	Dysentery	7 052	
0	Smallpox	0	
27 (6 under 1 year)	Measles	132 088	(6752 under 1 year)
2	Acute poliomyelitis	5	
28	Acute encephalitis	44	
0	Post-encephalitis	36	
0	Malaria	33	
0	Food poisoning	2 340	
0	Leptospirosis	3	
0	Tetanus	6	
18	Infective jaundice	7 369	
11	Tuberculosis		
	Respiratory	994	(55 under 1 year)
	CNS including meningitis	39	
	Other forms	238	

8 deaths from chickenpox
102 deaths from meningococcal infection, 59 under 1 year

number of diphtheria and tetanus notifications must reflect the success of the methods used. The development of tissue typing may allow the identification of those who are most susceptible to serious sequelae.

This is not to say that the ideal has been reached. The smaller the numbers of infected children the larger looms the risk of iatrogenic disease. The whole programme needs to be constantly under review with figures of unimpeachable accuracy and with the most thorough individual examination of complications and sequelae which could be blamed on any part of the programme. Two features of current arrangements give this a particular importance. Firstly, policy decisions on the extent and the timing of the items included in the programme descend from specialist committees on to the doctors who accept and carry them out without any serious attempt at a critical appraisal. The doctor ceases to regard himself as having the ultimate responsibility for what he does or does not do for his patient, and this is never a wise arrangement.

Secondly, under a National Health Service, whose administration is responsible to parliament, any important decision may contain a political element and even an element derived from the personal experience of an influential minister. A prime minister whose own child has been damaged by post-vaccinial encephalitis could only with difficulty give a balanced judgement on a vaccination programme. Further, research into epidemiology or into the development of improved prophylactic techniques cannot really be conducted by the doctors who actually give the injections and who, in a resigned manner, do as they are bidden. The legal position of the doctor, who fails to follow the recommendations of the Department of Health and whose patient suffers a serious complication, has yet to be defined.

The existence of effective vaccination against rubella and mumps raises the question of additions to the programme.

Smallpox

The most dangerous of these diseases is smallpox, and as the first against which prophylaxis was applied it remains as it always has been the most controversial. No animal hosts are known so that the future eradication of the disease from the world is theoretically possible. Until then doctors, nurses, and all medical personnel who come into contact with patients could be regarded as somewhat foolish if they fail to accept vaccination and re-vaccination every three years. The same might be thought of travellers, of the armed forces, and of all those who service travellers coming from those countries where the disease remains endemic. Laboratory accidents with smallpox virus are possible.

Argument remains unresolved about the safest time for primary vaccination, particularly in countries like England and Wales where the disease is no longer endemic and where naturally the risk of serious complications of vaccination outweighs the risk of smallpox itself. Cerebral involvement within the first two years takes the form of an encephalopathy from which recovery is more likely to be complete than from the demyelinating encephalitis of older age groups. Post-vaccinial encephalitis still carries a mortality rate of 25 per cent and a high morbidity rate for neurological deficits in survivors. Vaccinia gangrenosa, which is not confined to primary vaccinations and has no exact relationship to measurable impairment of immunity production, responds favourably to immunotherapy and thiosemicarbazones; so also does eczema vaccinatum. Nevertheless the presence of eczema is regarded as an absolute contra-indication to vaccination. Generalized vaccinia is benign. Although the evidence against it is equivocal, vaccination of women during the first trimester of pregnancy is unwise.

Since, until smallpox has been eradicated from the world's population, vaccination will continue to be practised, efforts must be made to find strains of virus capable of stimulating immunity, but with reduced virulence. Meanwhile, Lane and Millar (1969) accepting a death rate of 1 per million primary vaccinations in the United States estimate that the vaccination of every baby for the next 30 years would cause 210 deaths. By limiting vaccination to travellers to endemic smallpox areas, military recruits and hospital staff, deaths would amount to 60. In England and Wales the risk is estimated as 2 deaths each year if every baby was vaccinated in the second year of life. This would have to be compared with the number of deaths that occur in an unprotected population as the result of contact with imported cases. The argument being unresolved, general practitioners and paediatricians must watch developments and statistical computations in an active and critical spirit.

Triple vaccine

Routine prophylaxis against diphtheria has been the safest and the most effective. Hypersensitivity is the chief complication, occurring mainly in adults and in children over the age of 12 years. Tetanus prophylaxis is not quite so effective partly because the patient's response is sometimes poor and the duration of protection may be relatively short. It is important that the booster doses recommended both on school entry and at school leaving should be carried out. Even with the amount of protection afforded by triple vaccine, whooping cough continues to hold an important place in the notifications of which there were 16 259 in

1971. More than half were for children under the age of 5 years and 6 per cent were in babies in the first 6 months of life when 20 of the 26 deaths occurred. In interpreting these apparent failures, the clinical nature of the diagnosis must be remembered. Not all paroxysmal cough is due to the specific pertussis bacillus. Pertussis vaccine fails to protect 15 per cent and successful immunization of 90 to 100 per cent of the child population seems necessary to prevent epidemics compared with only 66 per cent in the case of diphtheria. There is, too, the possibility that the pertussis component in the vaccine is responsible for the neurological complications which follow, reported as 1 in 50 000 in Sweden. Certainly pertussis need not be included in the booster doses, and recent exposés of some neurological disasters blamed on pertussis immunization have produced much parental unwillingness to accept pertussis in the primary immunization. The fact that such disasters complicate naturally occurring infectious diseases – unrealized by most parents – should not be forgotten by the doctor.

Poliomyelitis

The use of oral live attenuated virus gives good protection and appears to be safe. Although the virus multiplies in the intestine, giving local resistance to intestinal reinfection, and can be found in faeces for several weeks, no danger of spread appears to exist.

Measles

Measles notification in 1971 represented 73.6 per cent of all notifications in Table 15.1. The increased use of live attenuated measles virus in the second year of life must reduce the prevalence of the disease. The assumption can be reasonably made that the infants notified before their first birthday (5 per cent of the total) were infected from siblings and would therefore have been protected. The discovery that some forms of demyelinating brain disease now grouped as subacute sclerosing panencephalitis are due to measles virus makes protection of even greater importance and since measles has been a universal infection the possibility that the attenuated strains might produce the same sequelae as the wild virus would not be an argument against mass immunization. In fact such sequelae have not yet been reported (Dudgeon 1975).

Rubella

The main purpose of rubella immunization is to prevent fetal abnormalities and fetal and infant deaths. Manson and colleagues (1960) reported 9.5 per cent of fetal deaths (4.8 per cent controls), an infant mortality rate following rubella in the first trimester of 76.5 per 1000 live births (25.8 per 1000 controls). Major congenital defects affected 15.8 per cent. The range decreased from 60 per cent with exposure at one month to 5 per cent by the fourth month. Immunization is offered to girls of 11 to 14 years of age and to mothers, either sero-negative or with low haemagglutination-inhibiting antibodies (HAI), who are given the vaccine between the second and fourth days after delivery. The immunity appears long lasting.

Mumps

A live attenuated vaccine is being used in the United States, largely justified by the prevention of the orchitis found in 20 per cent of males infected after puberty. There is no plan to follow this example at present in England and Wales. There might be some value in making mumps a notifiable disease with reporting of complications so that a reasoned decision could be taken at some future date.

CHAPTER 16

Some system problems

(skeletal – cardiovascular – respiratory, including asthma – alimentary – urogenital, including enuresis)

SKELETAL (ORTHOPAEDIC PAEDIATRICS)

Many babies and children are treated either as in- or out-patients in orthopaedic departments. Nicholas Andry (1741) who coined the name 'orthopédie' was a French physician and the subject was 'preventing and correcting deformities of children'. The fact that the speciality is now practised by surgeons must not conceal the large non-surgical elements contained within it. The elaboration of operative techniques has made possible improvement of function, which is recognized as having priority over correction of deformity, while concern for the education and the emotional development of the child in the context of family life takes precedence even over surgical treatment. Still dominant is the aim of Robert Jones, to enable crippled children 'to become self-supporting citizens', and to give them 'far greater possibilities of activity and happiness'. The success of methods of prevention is shown by the decline in deformity from tuberculosis, osteomyelitis and acute anterior poliomyelitis. Nutritional rickets has been virtually eliminated from the white population (see Chapter 21). Accident surgery has meanwhile increased and so have the technical possibilities for the surgical treatment of cerebral palsy and congenital and developmental abnormalities of the limbs, particularly those associated with spina bifida and myelomeningocele (q.v.). Because of the more thorough surveillance of babies and of infants, doubts about the normality of hip joints and of feet have been stimulated. The NCB survey suggests a birth incidence of orthopaedic problems of 7.3 per 1000 (5700 in 1971) and a point prevalence at 7 years of 5.8 per 1000 (4600 in 1971). Among older children Perthes' disease and various forms of scoliosis and kyphosis, either of themselves or by reason of their treatment, are important causes of chronic handicap.

Many of the doubts to resolve which orthopaedic opinions are sought arise from 'abnormal' appearance rather than from defect of function. Parents and doctors readily attach anxiety to variations of the normal. Experience of these variations is essential. So, too, is a thorough understanding of motor development and of the ways in which restriction of freedom of movement and deprivation of sensory experience may hamper long-term progress, both physical and educational, besides causing frustration, boredom and emotional strain. Sharrard (1971) comments on 'the difficulty that many people have, laymen, doctors and orthopaedic surgeons included, in differentiating variation from the normal from significant deformity'. Few surgeons have time to observe normal babies in the newborn nursery.

Congenital dislocation and subluxation of the hip

Some babies are born with an established deformity due to dysplasia of the acetabulum or to muscular or neuro-muscular disorder (myelomeningocele or arthrogryposis). For the rest instability of the joint from laxity of the capsule may lead, if untreated, to secondary joint changes. Barlow's method of screening should reveal the majority of unstable hip joints. Even in the most experienced hands it will not reveal all. For example, tight adductors may prevent the characteristic reduction 'clunk'. A negative neonatal examination is not a final answer. Too often, when the diagnosis is made late, blame is attached to the initial neonatal examination, although the child has been examined by doctors at home and in clinics since birth, but the hip examination omitted. This is true when standing has been noted to be delayed. By contrast doubts raised by too early an examination may lead to unnecessary anxiety and treatment.

The incidence of positive screening tests is not the same as the incidence of congenital dislocation of the hips. The highest incidence of positive tests, 11 per 1000, is found on the first day of life and when one observer makes all the examinations on the population studied (Thieme *et al.* 1968). In half, stability of the joints as shown by a negative screening test was 'restored' after the third day of life. Barlow (1966) stated that 2.36 per cent of babies examined on the first day of life had an abnormal hip joint, but only 1 per cent when examined at one year of age. He considered that spontaneous recovery could occur within the first eight weeks of life.

The incidence in females is three to five times as great as in males. The estimated number of newborn babies affected in 1971 on Barlow's incidence is 18 500 (about 13 800 girls and 4600 boys). The amount of hospital time taken cannot be discerned in HIPE. If a reported incidence of unstable hips of 11 per 1000 live births be accepted, examination on the first day of life would have aroused suspicion in 8600 or one new baby every hour of every day during the year. Allowing that one half lose their abnormal signs within the first week, there would remain in the school population (5 to 14 years) some 40 000 children who either had been successfully treated or still had hip dislocation. In sharp contrast is the NCB figure for the 7-year-old prevalence, the result of a positive questionnaire medical history, of 1.1 per 1000, a point prevalence that would have produced 905 children, only 2.2 per cent of the expected number, if applied to the ten years of school life (5 to 14 years).

Notable clicks were found by Thieme and Wynne-Davies in 10 per cent of all 1881 consecutively delivered live born babies and laxity of the joint allowing abduction in the frog position to more than 90° in 6 per cent. It would appear that anxiety and perhaps orthopaedic consultation are only necessary when the characteristic reduction 'clunk' is felt and when it persists to the end of the first week of life. Finlay *et al.* (1967) who examined 14 594 consecutive live born babies within the first 36 hours of life found 60 with at least one dislocated or dislocatable hip after excluding neonatal deaths, babies with myelomeningocele and two with dislocations of 'teratological' (dysplasic) type. Although they noted that several had reduced the amount of laxity within 48 hours and thought that only 1 out of every 5 would remain abnormal otherwise, they recommended splinting for all. Their figure for incidence at birth was only 4 per 1000, the number of babies to be splinted in 1971 being estimated as 3132. It would be interesting to learn whether in a single year the actual number of babies so treated approximates to any of these figures. It would also be interesting to know whether abnormal findings at these early examinations bear any relation to the development of arthritis of the hip in later life.

There can be no doubt that screening examination of the hips is an important prophylactic procedure which should be generally taught and practised. The teaching should include the facts that certain types of dislocation do not respond to simple splinting, that dislocation can be missed at birth even by the most expert, and that re-examination of the hips should be included in surveillance assessments.

Congenital club foot (talipes equino-varus, talipes calcaneovalgus, metatarsus varus)

Many babies are born with their feet in the positions to which these names are given. In most the condition is bilateral and the full range of foot and ankle movements is possible or becomes possible within the first week of life. Any survey of incidence lacking precision in distinguishing true deformity from temporary positioning can only be misleading. Positional variations in the newborn do not necessarily require any other action than reassurance and possibly a later confirmatory examination. Ruth Wynne-Davies (1964) states that the chance of a baby having one of these conditions is 1 in 1000. McKeown and Record (1960) in Birmingham give a birth incidence of 4.4 per 1000 for talipes equinovarus alone. The NCB Survey produced a birth incidence of 4.1 per 1000 for 'club feet', 3.5 per cent of whom were stillborn or neonatal deaths with a 7 year prevalence of 3.1 per 1000 or 2570 seven-year-olds in 1971. The prevalence in the whole school population would have been about 24 000 As Wynne-Davies suggests that some forms of treatment do more harm than good it would seem that there is an urgent need for study. No doubt paediatricians and general practitioners have formed their own individual ways of selecting patients for orthopaedic consultation with a view to treatment. A controlled co-operative study in a stable population with the prospect of a long-term follow up should bring the desirable degree of certainty and might establish the characteristics of the normal adult foot with which the baby's foot should be encouraged to conform.

The experience in anaesthesia recently gained through neonatal surgery has encouraged earlier and more extensive tendon lengthening in severe talipes equinovarus with soft tissue release when the foot cannot be restored to a normal position by manipulation. Those who accept as the cause damage to the developing limb bud with consequent failure of the muscles to grow see the deformity as of long duration, seven months at the time of birth. As manipulation and pressure in the foot may damage the cartilaginous tarsal bones, the case for early surgery is a strong one especially as the ankle joint may remain mobile. Careful paediatric assessment of the young infant is an essential step, whether by a paediatrician or a paediatrically trained general practitioner, before any surgical operation is carried out. Congenital defects should be identified and the baby's fitness for anaesthetic and operation ensured.

Epiphyseal osteochondritis

A number of named conditions characterized by derangement of particular centres of ossification affect children mainly during the middle years of childhood.

One especially, Legge-Calvé-Perthes Syndrome (LCPS) or Perthes' disease of the upper femoral epiphysis, is important because of the interruption to life and education resulting from the commonly recommended immobilization treatment. An enquiry in April 1969 into the reasons for residence in long-stay hospitals in England and Wales found 12.3 per cent of the occupants (180 children out of a total of 1463) with the diagnosis of Perthes' disease, fractionally less than those with spina bifida, who were the commonest. This gives a prevalence among school children of 4.7 per 100 000 who are treated in hospital. Some are managed at home, so that this prevalence rate is likely to be an underestimate. Gough's figure for the United States, of between 10 and 100 for every 100 000 births (Gough 1954), would mean that about 800 potential sufferers are born each year, a number difficult to credit. The appearance of 80 fresh patients each year to add to those already under long-term treatment would produce a sizeable enough problem. But, whatever the size of the population, the need exists very carefully to review the validity of the practice of ordering periods of immobilization lasting for several years beyond the stage of acute symptoms.

The classification suggested by Catterall (1971) on which the treatment plan can be based allows a great reduction in the amount of immobilization of the patient, and the safety of this new approach has been confirmed by Kamhi and MacEwen (1975). Their aim, to create 'a favourable environment in which the disease process can run its course', should be applied not only to the position of the femoral head but also to the whole child. Prolonged immobilization, when it is essential, should be carried out under conditions which allow for education and development.

Scoliosis

So-called idiopathic scoliosis is a common finding in babies and in children. Ruth Wynne-Davies (1966, 68) studied 114 affected children in Edinburgh, and as controls a general population of 11 087 normal children aged 2 weeks to 18 years. She found two peaks of incidence, the first at less than one year of age and the second in later childhood. There were certain important differences between the two groups. With early onset the scoliosis was usually to the left, males predominated over females, 5 to 4, prevalence among close relatives was greater than in the general population, half resolved with treatment, half persisted and could become serious. The prevalence was 1.3 per 1000 ($n=3139$). With later onset the scoliosis was usually to the right, females predominated over males, 7 to 1, family history was more strongly positive and none recovered spontaneously. The prevalence was 1.8 per 1000 ($n=7894$). Both early and late onset scoliosis were found within one family.

Assuming a prevalence during school years of 1.8 per 1000 there would have been just under 14 000 children with scoliosis past and present in the school population in 1971. There would have been just over 1000 infants of less than one year of age, with persistence in 500 in spite of treatment. No special attempt to identify this group has been made in any of the population surveys.

The serious nature of severe kypho-scoliosis in its juvenile form cannot be gainsaid. Not only does it limit physical activity and growth, but in addition the bad cosmetic effect, particularly in girls, may easily affect the personality, outlook and attitude to life. Furthermore, attempts to control the condition by such devices as the Milwaukee brace or by spinal surgery themselves interfere with education. Present forms of treatment leave much to be desired. If early diagnosis can be followed by successful preventive treatment, this would seem still to be a neglected clinical area despite all that has been written about it by the orthopaedic surgeons (James 1967).

Health needs. Successful prevention rests on education and constant vigilance. At present the control of infections such as tuberculosis and anterior poliomyelitis is satisfactory and osteomyelitis has become rare. Modern dietary habits, vitamin enrichment of baby foods and the availability of vitamin D have all but eliminated the bone deformities of florid rickets. In all of these matters attention must be paid to immigrant populations whose traditions and whose possible differences in physical constitution may require special measures. For the prevention of accidents a much greater knowledge of aetiological factors is awaited.

Early recognition of orthopaedic defects depends on awareness of their physical signs, a more certain knowledge of the difference between true deformities and variations of the normal and the inclusion of an orthopaedic point of view in routine surveillance. The newborn period, the succeeding stages of motor development, school entry and the period of the growth spurt are times for careful observation.

A more thorough education in the common problems of the dislocatable hip, talipes, flat foot, knock knee, scoliosis and kyphosis, would allow the general practitioner and the paediatrician to relieve the orthopaedic out-patient departments of much unnecessary work. In exchange the orthopaedic surgeon should work closely with the centres which cater for children with cerebral palsy, with myelomeningocele and with other neurological deficits and diseases which are associated with dysfunction and deformity of joints.

In all this work the orthopaedic surgeon is supported by physiotherapists and hydrotherapy. Their importance is great both in preventive work and in habilitation when defect or deformity renders impossible the fulfilment of the normal programme of body control and motor development. The prosthetic bio-physicist and the limb fitter form part of the team. Their products are improving along with their educational standards. The elaboration of bio-medical equipment of all kinds should produce a demand for a degree course. The whole question of design, supply and maintenance of artificial limbs, calipers, hand-operated and electrical wheelchairs and other aids for independent living for the handicapped awaits a comprehensive solution. Delays in supply and in maintenance during the years of rapid growth have a deleterious effect on motivation and adaptability.

The section on long-stay hospitals contains much applicable to the care of the child with orthopaedic problems, including a discussion on the need to divide large institutions into family groups and the advisability of vesting control of the institution in an educationist rather than a doctor (see chapter 9).

The birth of children with congenital limb defects following thalidomide has drawn greater attention to the emotional and psychological effects of severe deformities. In the practice of orthopaedics from the moment when parents are told about and shown their baby, through childhood and into adolescence, these stresses and strains must always be remembered and parents and child be given every possible help to adjust to them.

CARDIOVASCULAR

Congenital malformations of the heart and great vessels provide the bulk of cardiovascular lesions in childhood. Rheumatic heart disease is discussed elsewhere. The calculation of incidence and prevalence is possible within certain limits only, in spite of much epidemiological study. Many reasons account for the difficulties. Firstly, not all children with anatomical abnormalities can be identified at birth or even within the early months of life. Secondly, functional murmurs and doubtful signs are plentiful and amounted to 26.3 per cent of patients in Hay's Liverpool study. These must be taken into account despite an absence of any pathological lesion, because many such babies need periodic cardiological observation before they can be dismissed as normal, and their parents need advice and reassurance if they are informed or become aware of the doctor's suspicions. The true incidence of actual anatomical abnormalities would be difficult to discover.

From the practical viewpoint, many newborn babies whose fetal circulations have been adequate fail to adjust to the establishment of pulmonary respiration. In 1971 there were 40 stillbirths with congenital anomalies of the circulatory system, 435 died in the first week, 104 on the first day. Medical needs are recognition and management of acute cardiac failure. That half of the affected babies die within the first year, 1260 in all in 1971, is generally accepted, although death may not be

Table 16.1. Hay (1966) 80 691 live born 1948–58

	RGSR 1971 deaths		*Diagnosed within first few months (6.3 per 1000)*	*Dead before Nov. 1965*	*Death rate age 7–17 (1.9 per 1000)*	*Percentage distribution of lesions*		*Hay's survey of Liverpool schools 5–14 130 936 children 1963 (2.2 per 1000)*		*Estimated population 1–14 yr 10 894 900 1971*
						at birth	*1965 2.8 per 1000*			
	0–14	0–1	*N*=510	*N*=153	per cent	*N*=376	*N*=223	*N*=291	per cent	*N*=38 950
VSD	304	226	128	21	16.4	34.0	48.0	82	28.1	10 945
PDA	45	41	29	10	34.5	7.7	8.5	41	14.1	5 492
ASD	122	96	44	20	45.5	11.7	10.8	44	15.1	5 881
AV canal	23	18								
Coarctation	62	57	20	11	55.0	5.3	4.0	7	2.5	974
Fallot	135	40	22	15	15.0	5.9	3.1	11	3.8	1 480
Aortic stenosis	10	9	16	3	18.8	4.2	5.8	34	11.7	4 557
Pulmonary artery stenosis and			{30	2	6.6	8.0	12.6	51	17.5	6 816
atresia	40	27	{10	8	80.0	2.7	0.9	1		
Transposition	189	139	21	18	85.7	5.6	1.3	2		
Common truncus	49	46	6	5	83.3	1.6	0.5	0	1.4	545
Tricuspid atresia	not separated		45	45	80.0	1.3	0.5	1		
Others*	686	561	—			12.0	4.0	17	5.8	2 260
Total	1665	1260				100.0	100.0	291	100.0	38 950
Functional systolic murmur			79							
Doubtful			55							

*Anomalies of		
great veins	26	25
heart valves	137	108
Fibroelastosis cordis	68	58
Other lesions specified	[illegible]	[illegible]

directly due to the heart lesion, but to some complication or an acute infection.

Prevalence in the school population is also difficult to calculate, partly because of uncertainty of diagnosis. Hay's study in Liverpool (Table 16.1) gave 2.8 per 1000 in his follow up of babies born in 1948 to 1958 when they were examined in 1965, while a survey of the total Liverpool school population in 1963 gave 2.2 per 1000. The difference in survival rates is reflected in the change in the percentages of the individual heart lesions in infancy compared with those at school age.

The 1958 Cohort studied by the National Children's Bureau began with a birth incidence of 7 per 1000 total (not only live) births, which had fallen to a 7-year-old prevalence of 3.5 per 1000, 1.7 per 1000 reported as seriously affected. In the Isle of Wight Study the 10- to 12-year-old prevalence was 2.4 per 1000. Maurice Campbell (Watson 1968) surveying the literature arrived at a birth incidence of 6 per 1000 (range 4.2–8.5). For the present purpose, 6.5 per 1000 live births is adopted as birth incidence and 3 per 1000 as the prevalence in the school population.

The development of cardiac surgery may well be altering the prevalence rate. Before this can produce a practical change great improvement in both surgical and medical management of babies in their first year will be needed as well as more effective case finding and more widely available expertise.

Deaths from congenital malformations of the cardiovascular system 0–14 in 1971 (RGSR) amounted to 1665 of which 104 died on the first day, 435 in the first week, 284 in the ensuing three weeks and a total of 1260 had died by the end of the first year. With an estimated 5090 live born affected babies, 3830 are presumed to be surviving at the end of the first year. This 75 per cent apparent survival contrasts with the 50 per cent consistently found in special surveys and suggests that many of the deaths are recorded in RGSR under other headings, such as acute respiratory disease, rather than that the incidence rate is wide of the mark. If 3 per 1000 is accepted for prevalence in the school population 5–14 years, the number in 1971 should have been 23 270 to which must be added the 1–4-year group (estimated 4 per 1000) of 15 680, a total of 38 950. Estimates of numbers with the commoner abnormalities in the population in 1971 aged 1–14 years form the last column in Table 16.1. Of these, applying the NCB estimate that 1.7 per 1000 at 7 years are seriously affected, some 14 000 children should have been needing treatment for clinical symptoms during the year (approximate number of 7-year-olds = 825 000 in 1971).

Prevention. Prevention is considered under two separate headings, the prevention of maldevelopment of the heart and the prevention of unnecessary invalidism. *Rubella* is the most important known aetiological agent and some reduction of birth incidence should follow rubella immunization. Higgins (1965) found the two main lesions accountable to fetal rubella to be persistent ductus arteriosus (58.1 per cent) and ventricular septal defect (17.6 per cent) with Fallot's tetralogy next (7.2 per cent) and all the other lesions amounting to 17.1 per cent. In general, no study has shown a significant variation between the sexes, ethnic groups or socio-economic status (Morton *et al.* 1966, Higgins, 1965). Coarctation of the aorta is, in fact, commoner in males and persistence of the ductus arteriosus in females.

Some chromosomal abnormalities are associated with heart lesions, and the identification and termination of such pregnancies would reduce numbers. One example is the persistent ostium atrio-ventriculare commune in the mongol.

Linde and colleagues (1966) have discussed attitudinal factors concluding that maternal anxiety is due to the presence rather than the severity of the lesion. Maternal protectiveness, arising from anxiety and guilt, led to pampering and was met by aggressive, attention-seeking dependence. Failure of the child to adjust could also cause a passive physical dependence with considerable anxiety and the use of 'illness' to secure 'secondary gains'. Unnecessary restriction of physical activity hampers development and warps character.

Health needs. The life history of the child affected by congenital heart disease or suspected on account of abnormal physical signs will determine the nature of his medical care. The majority will come under paediatric care in the neonatal period. Many will require emergency treatment for heart failure and those who survive will need careful follow up including accurate assessment and diagnosis of the anatomical lesion.

Expert paediatric cardiology will be wise for the most severely affected and palliative or corrective surgery where this is appropriate. If it be true that each annual cohort loses half its numbers by the end of the first year, there should be between 2000 and 3000 left. Although the age for operation varies for different lesions, in a population that has achieved a 'steady state' of cardiac surgery, each year could see the demand for operation in about 400 children with persistent ductus, 50 or 60 with coarctation, 80 with Fallot's tetralogy. A proportion of septal defect cases would need repair and each year would add some 800 ventricular and 400 atrial septal defects. There is no doubt that some of the former close spontaneously. Using the Liverpool figures about 300 babies are expected each year with transposition so that, if the Rashkind procedure were completely successful, this number would be added each year to the school population.

In the whole school population, about 14 000 children at any one time would be in need of careful supervision for more or less severe symptoms. There remain 25 000 for some of whom routine supervision should be adequately provided in paediatric departments on the basis of a visit every year or every other year, and for others by the general practitioner. In fact the number of school children requiring treatment and/or observation for heart conditions in England and Wales in 1969 was 30 752. This fits reasonably well with the estimated numbers.

The establishment of specialist paediatric cardiological clinics in every region is certainly justified by numbers. Yet congenital cardiovascular anomalies are so widely distributed in the population that all who have clinical care of children must be required to have the skill not only to recognize and manage the commonest conditions, but also to recognize when more expertise is needed. For children with disabling lesions who await assessment and possible operation and who are unfit for day school, educational requirements should be filled by home tutors and only when home and family are unable to contain the problem should the child be housed in a residential school. The fortitude demanded of the child undergoing investigation and surgical treatment for cardiovascular anomaly is best established in the security of home and family. This presupposes a home and family secure and stable, both physically and emotionally.

RESPIRATORY SYSTEM

The respiratory tract occupies a dominant position in medical practice. Its diseases and disorders provide almost one quarter of hospital paediatric in-patient practice (HIPE) and about 55 per cent of general practitioner childhood consultations (GPR). The severe congenital defects, notably pulmonary agenesis, are incompatible with life, premature fetal respiratory efforts may place in jeopardy the integrity of the brain or life itself, but during childhood the system provides the seat of recurrent infection and of the expression of allergy and of emotional stress. The state of the system and the expectation of how it will respond are the frequent concerns of almost every doctor whatever form of medicine he practises.

Yet knowledge is still lacking in many of the most important particulars. Before the era of antibiotics, the skin, the umbilical cord and the conjunctiva provided important sites on which the newborn baby could test its power to control invading bacteria. There were casualties which modern treatment has reduced to vanishing point. Efficient prophylaxis together with the improved hygiene of milk, which now largely protects the infant's alimentary tract from pathogens, has left the respiratory epithelium as the main proving ground of the competence of the new baby to defend itself against bacteria, since complete respiratory prophylaxis in the normal world is unattainable. Clinically the distinction between viral and bacillary illness remains as confusing as the separation of the allergic element from the rest of the symptomatic response to infection. What part antibiotics should play in treatment is always difficult to assess. Does their too ready or too early use impede the production of the immunity which could protect from further infection? The answer is no easier to give to this than to the other major questions, what part is played by tonsils and adenoid tissue in the process of immunity and on what precise grounds and when should this lymphoid tissue be removed?

Parental anxiety over the early evidences of respiratory disease and a lack of tolerance for any rise in body temperature produce an irresistible pressure upon the doctor. The younger the doctor the more difficult is it for him to withstand such pressure. His pattern of response to respiratory symptoms tends to become fixed and when experience eventually makes him a more authoritarian figure, his wish to husband antibiotic resources only for use in serious bacterial infections may have evaporated.

Figures are given in Chapters 10 and 11 for the amount of hospital and general practitioner work in the treatment of acute respiratory disease. Obviously much upper respiratory infection including 'the common cold' is handled by parents at home without the aid of the doctor. Pneumonia commands more medical attention although much is now treated at home by the general practitioner. The tendency observed in Newcastle (Miller *et al.* 1974) is for lower respiratory infection to be commonest in the first year, slowly declining until school. An increase in recurrent upper respiratory infection follows school entry and during school years upper respiratory tract infections predominate. Until effective prophylaxis or some general and generally available antiviral agent has been developed, respiratory tract disorders, acute and chronic will continue to make great demands on medical time.

Were respiratory tract diseases and disorders rare, controlled observations by research-minded physicians would probably have led to valid answers to many of the questions. As it is, the very size of the clinical opportunities has made research too formidable a task. Here is an ideal subject for the general practitioner to study in a stable community of families. Epidemiology, aetiology, the importance of home hygiene, the effectiveness of drug treatment, the careful analysis of accurately observed signs and symptoms, the factors that predispose to recurrence and above all the long-term effect of surgical treatment on life history. All these and many more illuminations are required. Meanwhile medical training should reinstate clinical study. What parents call a cold, now too often dutifully transcribed by the doctor in his notes, can be anything from an unilateral purulent nasal discharge due to a button in a nostril to the allergic reaction of the nasal mucosa at the onset of an attack of asthma. When 'recurrent colds' provide the excuse for a consultation with the oto-rhino-laryngologist with a view to removal of tonsils and adenoids, the paediatrician is bypassed. This would matter less if these specialists had been trained in paediatrics. Until that time arrives, the normal large tonsils of the pre-school child will continue to be miscalled 'enlarged tonsils' and hospital beds will continue to be misused for the surgical treatment of what is called 'hypertrophy of tonsils and adenoids'.

Asthma

The only chronic and recurring conditions of the respiratory tract of numerical importance are those due wholly or in part to allergy and are discussed under the generic title of asthma. The asthmatic child is more easily recognized than defined. Inasmuch as asthma is a symptom with a variable and multi-factorial aetiology, incidence and prevalence have an artificiality which has discouraged careful epidemiological study. In the Isle of Wight assessment, a child was counted among asthmatics who had had at least one attack of breathlessness with audible wheezing in the year preceding the survey. The prevalence rate at 10 to 12 years of age was 23.2 per 1000. The NCB study, accepting a mother's statement that her 7-year-old had at some time had one or more attacks of asthma, found a prevalence of 3.1 per cent with a slight preponderance of boys over girls (3.8 to 2.3 per cent). That the prevalence was almost twice as high in social Class I as in social Class V suggests that research here may elucidate some provocative factors.

J. M. Smith (1961) surveyed Birmingham school children and found a prevalence rate of only 17.6 per 1000 (boys 23.1 and girls 11.7) noting that boys had less trouble as age advanced while the rate in girls remained steady. On the other hand, Dawson *et al.* (1967), who included pre-school children, gave the figure of 48 per 1000 with an onset before age 5 years in 81 per cent. They found the majority of mild cases in the non-manual classes.

The Newcastle group appears studiously to avoid the term asthma, preferring 'recurrent wheezing disease' even when associated with eczema. The HIPE (1971) discharges credited to asthma numbered 12 335 and there is little doubt that many of the younger children, labelled as unspecified pneumonia and bronchitis, should be included in the group. Whatever title is employed, no-one would deny that episodes of wheezy breathing of asthmatic type diminish in frequency during childhood, at least in boys. Assuming a prevalence rate of 3 per cent from 1–14 years (n = 11 676 500), some 350 000 children have asthmatic attacks each year. The number of school children requiring treatment and/or observation for lung conditions during 1969 is recorded as 51 168.

Whatever his sufferings are called the 'asthmatic child' has many health needs. The majority of the children can be adequately handled by the general practitioner who can secure symptomatic relief without a full diagnosis of all the contributory factors. The present predilection for assessment would lead to an early and complete study of any child with recurrent attacks of respiratory illness which interfere with family or school life. Into the assessment would enter, besides studies of lung function and lung structure, a search for allergens, tests for immunoglobulins (Ig E) and for the presence of disease in the upper respiratory tract, psychometric and psychiatric explorations, and studies of the family, the home and the socio-economic environment. Unfortunately, asthmatic symptoms thrive on anxiety and such a programme might be more harmful to child and parents than advice about minimizing the effect which the recurrent symptoms have on life at home and at school and the prescription of appropriate drugs. These decisions are properly made by the general practitioner in concert, if necessary, with the paediatrician. Unfortunately, many asthmatic children are separated from Departments of Child Health because the view is taken that specific allergens are probably involved and that reference should be made to a department of Allergy which is not necessarily paediatric in outlook. The compulsion of the general practitioner to have an x-ray report on the child's lungs leads to a 'chest clinic' where one advantage is that the chest x-ray is almost a prerequisite for attendance. Here, too, a paediatric outlook may be missing. Parents of asthmatic children are often biased towards multiple consultations, a bias which is encouraged by these approaches and which may not always be beneficial. This is not to deny that many allergy clinics and some chest clinics do furnish effective treatment.

Careful case selection should be the answer. It is not only the severity or the frequency of the attacks, but their effect on the emotions and on the lives of the members of the family that should lead to full assessment. Such an assessment takes a long time, always more than one consultation and often more than one consultant. In the hospital, recurrent respiratory disease is entitled to as elaborate a team approach as congenital heart disease or spina bifida even although surgery is seldom required. Only in this way can integrated treatment become available and splintered treatment be avoided.

Under the title of asthma are included all degrees of illness from the eczematous baby whose one or two attacks of wheezy bronchitis in the second year of life may yield to encouraging words and suitable drugs, to the child in status asthmaticus who needs all the facilities of the intensive care unit. Accurate quantification of need is impossible. But the application of Dawson's Aberdeen results (1967) to the estimated 350 000 asthmatic children would produce 57 750 severely affected (16.5 per cent) with ten or more attacks in a year and without full recovery between, a figure compatible with the total of school children requiring treatment and/or observation for a lung condition (51 168), most of whom would be 'chesty' asthmatics, 147 700 of moderate severity (42.2 per cent) and 144 550 mildly affected (41.3 per cent) with 1 to 5 yearly attacks and complete recovery between.

Paediatric out-patient departments should certainly contain one organisation that can handle the total problem, and a sound knowledge of all that is involved in 'asthma' in childhood should be imparted at the undergraduate stage.

ALIMENTARY TRACT

The detailed discussion of these conditions seems more appropriate here than in the general chapter on hospital admission under Class IX.

Appendicitis and appendicectomy. Criteria for the diagnosis of acute appendicitis and Sir Frederick Treves' operation for appendicectomy (1888) have become textbook stereotypes. The appendix problem is regarded as settled. In 1886, Reginald Fitz of Boston had first suggested surgical treatment for the appendix abscess and in 1887, T. G. Morton (1888) successfully removed the perforated appendix as part of this procedure. It was only a short step to perform appendicectomy for 'relapsing typhlitis' and then for the acute inflammation that might be leading to perforation and abscess formation. Treves himself (1888) had written 'if by some magic process an attack of typhlitis could be foretold, it could be prevented in a large proportion of cases by a removal of the appendix itself . . .'. So, with another short step and bearing in mind all the anxiety generated by the dangers of the perforated appendix lying in a pool of pus, the surgeon has transferred some of his intervention to the child with acute or recurrent abdominal pain, unconcerned whether this be therapy or prophylaxis.

The relief which has followed the surgeon's ability to save life by a simple operation, followed by all the improvements in anaesthesia and in pre- and post-operative care and by the use of antibiotics, appears to have paralysed further thinking. HIPE records 29 044 discharges and deaths of children with appendicitis. The facts that about 80 children have the appendix removed in one or other hospital in England and Wales every single day of the year, and that despite this during 1971 31 children (one child about every 12 days) were registered as dying, 24 with peritonitis, are accepted as inevitable. Is this important enough by reason of suffering, anxiety, ill health, interruption to education or cost to the health service to merit a special study?

Is appendicitis preventable? Is the diagnosis accurately made in the maximum possible number of cases? Is the operation always necessary, that is to say is *appendicectomy* sometimes preventable? What are the reasons for failure to diagnose or for the loss of life that remains in the record?

Certain special attitudes of mind can be discerned in the medical profession and certain unusual procedures which deserve study. First is the commonly held belief that recurrent abdominal pain in children can be caused by a 'grumbling' or 'chronically inflamed appendix'. Second is the idea that when, in such a case, the normal appendix is found, it should be removed on the grounds that human beings are better and safer without this vestigial organ. Third is the practice of not regarding this episode as a 'mistake', but as a positive benefit, a practice which inevitably leads to carelessness in diagnosis. And fourthly, the habit of morbid anatomists of failing to report a normal appendix when the normal organ and the sections are examined. A generous verdict all too often supplied for the surgeon is of 'early inflammatory changes'.

Most paediatricians would agree that children do not have 'grumbling' appendices. The failure of the surgeon to acknowledge a diagnostic error can lead to the failure of a correct diagnosis, such as a urinary infection or even an inflamed Meckel's diverticulum. The 'better out than in' concept not only confirms parents in their fear of appendicitis which contributes to anxiety and tension when the child complains of recurrent abdominal pain but would lead logically to the inference that every child should have his appendix removed at some selected age. Inexact criteria provide one of the reasons for the failure of correct diagnosis which leads to perforation, peritonitis and death. Another is still, of course, delayed referral by parents.

A survey is needed which would include a study of admission procedures for children sent by general practitioners to hospital with 'acute abdominal pain, query appendicitis'. Accurately to examine young and frightened children in the casualty department is impossible. All should be admitted, pacified, settled in their warm beds, and examined slowly and quietly for tenderness, resistance and the rest. A common routine is for premedication to be given and arrangements with anaesthetists and operating theatres to be made from Casualty. The question needs an answer, why is there such great urgency? This urgency contrasts with the somewhat slow approach to the treatment of intussusception, where there is a real emergency, and which caused 25 deaths in the first year of life, with another 3 deaths in older children (1971).

Mason Brown (1956) reporting from the Royal Hospital for Sick Children, Edinburgh, analyzed the 263 children admitted with 'acute appendicitis' in 1952. In 151 diagnosis was confirmed at operation. He does not record whether by clinical or histological examination. Of the remaining 112, 73 were later diagnosed as having probable or definite mesenteric adenitis, 16 of the latter were appendicectomized. The appendix was removed in another 8, the only 3 with primary peritonitis, 2 when nothing abnormal was found, and one each for pneumonia, Meckel's diverticulitis, torsion of the omentum and thread worms in the appendix. 'In none of these is it (removal) an error.' Under the very good conditions of a children's hospital with staff experienced in examining children, Mason Brown accepted that the clinical diagnosis in older children would prove wrong in 2.4 per cent. 'Provided that this does not happen with undue frequency it should be regarded as the insurance premium which is paid lest some serious catastrophe arise, rather than an error for which junior members of a team should be taken to task'. This would have meant the removal of a normal appendix from some 700 children in 1971, and more unless the standard of care is assumed to have been as high as all NHS hospitals as in the Edinburgh Sick Children's. When no paediatric surgeon is available, nothing would be lost and much might be gained by referring children under suspicion of acute appendicitis to the paediatrician. This should be the routine method when the condition is believed to be chronic.

Hernia and intestinal obstruction

Morbidity and more especially mortality from what are essentially mechanical defects should be treatable although some of the defects are lethal in the newborn. In the rest success depends upon the avoidance of complications and this in turn depends upon early recognition of the defect and informed clinical observation. Inguinal hernia without mention of obstruction accounted for 16 599 discharges and no deaths are recorded, inguinal hernia with obstruction numbered 1439 with 13 deaths. Of other hernias of the abdominal cavity without mention of obstruction there were 3931 and 133 deaths and with obstruction 144 and 8 deaths.

The deaths occurred mainly in patients with either diaphragmatic (94) or umbilical hernias (43). Most of the former (74) died on the first day and another 15 within the first week, presumably the condition being impossible or extremely difficult to repair. Similarly all but seven of the deaths from umbilical hernia are recorded in the first month and seem likely to have been of babies with exomphalos, which like diaphragmatic hernia is not mentioned under congenital defects (Class XIV).

It must be regretted that as many as 82 children died of 'intestinal obstruction without mention of hernia', a group the main components of which are intussusception (28) and volvulus (21). Unspecified obstruction accounts for a further 25. During the first year there were 25 deaths from intussusception and 17 from volvulus. There is no way of determining the numbers of children with these conditions who were successfully treated nor whether there is any difference in results between general and paediatric surgeons or in general or paediatric hospitals and units. With regard to the newborn babies born in hospital, selection of a special centre should now be possible in most parts of the United Kingdom, a matter discussed under Malformations. With other children the doctor of primary care is faced with an emergency, speed is paramount and the referral would be largely dictated by geography and transport. The early recognition of intestinal obstruction and of peritonitis in babies and young children, with their life-saving content, must always be important teaching subjects.

Other conditions

A small toll of 69 deaths was taken by a number of conditions listed below (Table 16.2) the deaths reported in RGSR being related in the table to the HIPE discharges and deaths. The two largest HIPE groups could furnish interesting information about the conduct of investigation and treatment of children with digestive disturbances, were subdivisions

Table 16.2. Some other conditions in the alimentary tract

ICD		*HIPE*	*RGSR deaths*
530	Diseases of the oesophagus	399	19
531–3	Peptic ulceration	277	7
561	Gastro-enteritis		
	non infectious	1506	3
563	Ulcerative colitis	376	7
567	Peritonitis	188	11
570-7	Diseases of liver and gall bladder	321	22
570	hepatic necrosis	11	2
571	cirrhosis	133	11
565	Anal fissure and abscess	1030	0
564	Functional disorders of intestine	5470	0

and full diagnosis recorded. 'Functional disorders of the intestine' (5470) and gastro-enteritis and colitis, except ulcerative, of non-infectious origin' (376) undoubtedly include some very important conditions. In Class XVI we shall meet 'symptoms referable to abdomen and lower gastro-intestinal tract' to the number of 18 935 discharges (no deaths). Taken together these total 24 781 and the question arises as to whether admission to hospital might have been avoided if facilities for out-patient investigation were sufficiently well organized.

The picture of alimentary tract disease presented by the General Practitioner Survey of 53 practices is very different. The class total (ICD 520–577) amounts to 2947, but almost half of this (1320) concerns teeth, jaws, oral cavity and salivary glands. There were 24 patients with peptic ulceration (ICD 531–3) and 231 with functional disorders of stomach (ICD 536). Appendicitis (ICD 540–3) is recorded in 181 and hernia (ICD 550–3) in 222. Constipation accounted for 487 patient consultations and it would be valuable to know the criteria of diagnosis. In 407 diagnosis was incomplete.

The same incompleteness marks the large number of 5321 with abdominal problems in the class labelled 'symptoms and ill-defined conditions' (XVI-ICD 780–796). The largest number is 3602 'acute vomiting and/or diarrhoea'. Abdominal pain is variously categorized as colic 716, appendicular pain 86 and 'other non-colicky' pain 767. Anorexia was the reason for 101 patients consulting; it is probable that disorders of appetite were present in many more of the children. Food refusal and bad mealtime behaviour are extremely common in the under-5-year-olds. The fact that it is so often not the presenting symptom does not lessen its importance in the causation of other alimentary symptoms, especially abdominal pain, and of other and more general symptoms. This is a subject the teaching of which is of the utmost importance (see Chapter 3).

UROGENITAL

Growing importance attaches to disorders of the urinary tract since diagnostic methods have become more sophisticated, treatment more effective and most recently renal dialysis and transplantation have become available. These changes provide the basis for a speciality of paediatric nephrology.

At the level of common practice lie three problems, large in dimensions, first that of lack of control of micturition and then the problems in boys of circumcision and in girls of bacteriuria. Whatever the truth of the matter, these three problems are related to each other in the minds, not only of parents and school teachers, but also of the doctors. Much remains to be learned.

Although some children are admitted to hospital for the observation and investigation of enuresis, the condition is not identifiable in HIPE. True enuresis or the inappropriate voiding of urine by an involuntary act of micturition has to be distinguished from the various forms of true incontinence by careful history taking and observation. The distinction can be made in the early months of life even by parents, provided they realize that constant dribbling wetness differs from involuntary acts of micturition. The natural history of the development of micturition control should be part of health education as well as of undergraduate instruction.

Questionnaire studies are expected to yield greater numbers than those known to doctors, since some families are very tolerant. Miller *et al.* (1960) found that only one third of the children who wet the bed after the age of 10 years had been taken to the doctor. This is fortunate as some 88 000 10-year-old children alone are expected still to lack control of micturition at night in England and Wales. For other parents failure of the child to gain control by night at the age of two years causes intense anxiety. Both NCB and Newcastle surveys agree that about 11 per cent of children wet the bed between the ages of 5 and 11 years. The latter differentiated three groups of children, the largest being 5-year-olds, who have never been dry; some had been dry but had relapsed and a few became dry after 5 years only to relapse later. These facts are not surprising when enuresis is accepted as the result of stress from adverse social, emotional and intellectual factors leading to failure to mature or to regression of behaviour towards a less mature stage. The doctor's responsibility is to help the family to steer an accurate course between neglect and unnecessary investigation and treatment. Kolvin *et al.* (1973)

have brought together the results of much modern research and thinking. Careful history taking, a meticulous examination and insight into family relationships should enable the general practitioner to select those families whose affected child needs detailed study. There are always emotional reactions in all parties concerned, sometimes including the doctor, but as an isolated symptom enuresis is rarely psychogenic in origin. When lack of control is regarded by adults or peers as wrong or bad, the emotional effects on the child, his self esteem and his behaviour have to be borne in mind and may be serious enough to perpetuate the condition.

The problem of circumcision has been discussed in Chapter 10 and the high proportion of operations on boys in the 5- to 14-year-age group was noted. A group of parents exists who feel an uncontrollable need to submit one of their children to some surgical operation (Franklin 1960). An investigation is overdue into the extent to which this need contributes to such a medically acceptable procedure as circumcision as well as to removal of tonsils, adenoids and appendix. There is no evidence that circumcision plays a part in the management of the enuretic boy, although this is a question posed by some parents.

During 1971 what was referred to as a redundant prepuce or phimosis led to about 20 000 circumcisions, hypertrophy of tonsils to 96 000 tonsillectomies, and 29 000 appendices were removed. These operations account for 145 000 discharges during the year, 16.8 per cent of the total and approximately the same proportion as result from accidents of all kinds. Many of the operations were performed on young children and may have caused the first separation from home and family. Paediatricians are not always summoned to give advice on these 'common or garden' matters. The indications for surgical intervention are ill-defined. Anxiety, lack of confidence, the temptation to act or recommend action rather than inaction, all play some part in the doctor's mind when he makes his decision. A co-ordinated survey into the circumstances, clinical, pathological, emotional and social, surrounding one or more circumscribed populations and an attempt at some form of controlled follow-up, might well enable medical teachers to present a more rational account to undergraduates. On-going computer-based diagnosis has already been shown to reduce the number of appendicectomies in one group of hospitals (de Dombal *et al.* 1975). The natural history of the foreskin and reactions of human beings to its presence and its removal still need much serious study.

Urinary tract infections are sometimes present in enuretic girls. The possibility that untreated chronic or recurrent urinary infections with ureteric reflux contribute to chronic renal disease, pyelitis of pregnancy and perhaps the later development of hypertension, has led to the devising of screening methods and these have been applied to schoolgirl populations. That such screening methods lead to the finding of undiagnosed lower urinary tract infection has now been amply proved (Meadow *et al.* 1969; Savage *et al.* 1973; Newcastle ASB Research Group 1975). Prevalence of bacteriuria among girls at school entry varies between 1.4 to 1.6 per cent and rises, from 7 to 11 years, to over 2.0 per cent. Asymptomatic or covert bacteriuria are names now applied to positive test results, the latter name because close questioning reveals that although parents failed to seek medical advice, symptoms were often present.

In the Newcastle series, these were urgency (39 per cent), abdominal pain (31 per cent), and nocturnal enuresis (30 per cent), the last being the only symptom with a significant correlation with the presence of renal scarring or ureteric reflux. There was no evidence to support the idea of progressive renal damage during childhood. While the Newcastle group agrees with the Dundee group (Savage *et al.* 1973) that the case for prescriptive screening of schoolgirls has not been made, these studies reveal a well of undiagnosed and therefore untreated urinary tract infections in girls which are associated with symptoms. The subject, therefore, seems of importance in teaching while further experience of the effectiveness of treatment in eliminating the bacteria and relieving symptoms is awaited. The estimated number of schoolgirls with 'asymptomatic' or covert bacteriuria in England and Wales at any one time is about 56 650. Applying the Newcastle results 8500 would show radiological scarring, 22 000 would suffer from urgency of micturition, 17 500 from abdominal pain (not necessarily due to the bacteriuria), and nearly 17 000 would wet the bed. The prevalence of bacteriuria in boys from 5 to 18 years was only 0.2 per cent, which represents a mere 80 boys. Since nocturnal enuresis is slightly more common among boys than girls, these estimates lend little support to the importance of the bacteriuria in the aetiology of nocturnal enuresis.

Doctors are faced with the need to advise on these three problems, the need for circumcision, the need for and the 'best' methods of sphincter training and of treating the child who wets the bed and the diagnosis and treatment of so-called 'cystitis' and infection of the lower urinary tract. Even today because of a general absence of scientifically established fact, despite the many studies, the advice tends to be arbitrary and based on prejudices, tradition and habit.

Taken more seriously are the children with acute nephritis who are encountered relatively frequently. Some remain at home in the hands of the doctor of primary care, some reach hospital beds for all or for some part of their management. Chronic nephritis and the nephrotic syndrome have attracted much study to which improved renal biopsy methods, improved experience of histological interpretation, and identification of patterns of amino-acid excretion have contributed much. These conditions remain serious in morbidity and mortality and, having played their part in illuminating problems of renal physiology and pathology, hold deservedly an important place in hospital medicine. The haemolytic-uraemic syndrome can require the assistance of a renal dialysis unit, although the textbooks include it in diseases of the blood. The prevalence appears to be increasing. No quantitative estimate is possible for these 'medical' diseases involving the kidneys. All are likely to require hospital paediatrics.

Centres for the practice of paediatric nephrology would need to be closely associated with adult departments. A special interest in all problems of the urinary tract should allow of better teaching and training. The BPA has accepted the figure of 3 to 4 per million population of annual deaths from chronic renal disease in children from birth to age 15 years. In 1971 this should have produced between 146 and 195 deaths. As the Association suspected, this is a low estimate, and RGSR records during the year no less than 262 deaths, of whom 154 had congenital defects, 92 of whom died during the first week of life, presumably many with renal agenesis of which 90 would have been anticipated (incidence 2 per million population). These would only be chronic in terms of fetal life. Unfortunately pulmonary hypoplasia is a frequent concomitant of renal agenesis. Polycystic and multicystic kidneys accounted for 24 deaths in the first week and a further 7 by the end of the first year.

All these congenital defects are judged to be acceptable for possible renal transplantation (BPA Council Report) along with chronic bilateral pyelonephritis when bladder and urethra are normal either naturally or after surgical operation, non-active glomerulo-nephritis and bilateral renal calculi without metabolic abnormality. A supply of neonatal kidneys would require special organization. The view was taken that there was no place for long term haemodialysis except as a prelude to renal transplantation.

Renal neoplasms are considered in Chapter 17. The supervision of treatment and the follow-up require the complex oncology team and need to be based on hospital. Early diagnosis is the prerequisite for success. The doctor of primary care should familiarize himself with the techniques of clinical examination of the abdomen in infants and young children, even although it may never fall to his lot to find a renal enlargement.

Other congenital defects than renal agenesis or polycystic kidneys are associated with dilatation of the renal pelvis and ureters. Ectopia vesicae presents major problems for urologist, plastic surgeon and child psychiatrist.

Although numbers are comparatively small (see Table 10.3), the specialty of paediatric urologist is of great value. His expertise can be communicated to general paediatric surgeons or in other geographical areas to the urologist for adults. The centralization of patients into specialist clinics enlarges knowledge and benefits individual patients.

CHAPTER 17

Some special diseases

(diabetes mellitus – cystic fibrosis – adrenogenital syndrome – haemophilia – muscular dystrophy – malignancy)

DIABETES MELLITUS

Juvenile diabetes, according to Joslin, accounts for between 10 and 14 per cent of the total diabetic population. Sterky in Sweden (1963) found that among the 79 658 school children in Stockholm, there were 115 diabetic children aged 7 to 14 years, giving a prevalence rate of 1.44 per 1000. In 1971 in England and Wales this age group contained 6 121 100 children, so that the expected number of diabetic children would have been 8814. Hubble (1969) gives a prevalence under 5 years of 0.3 per 1000 and of 1 per 1000 during the school years, or 8932 children under 15 in 1971. Bloom *et al.* (1975) have estimated a minimum yearly incidence of 7.67 newly diagnosed diabetic children per 100 000, which gives 895 fresh children in 1971 ignoring the sex difference. RGSR records 25 deaths from diabetes mellitus during the year, 4 before the first and 9 before the fifth birthday. There were 5171 discharges and deaths in HIPE. The size of the contribution to perinatal death and morbidity made by maternal diabetes is unknown.

Sterky investigated the background of his patients and using a matched non-diabetic control group looked for any adverse effect on the diabetic children's school life. The mean age of onset was 7 years and the median duration of the disease 5½ years at the time of the study. The socio-economic background matched the usual pattern in Stockholm and school achievement matched the controls. In general there was no bias towards maladjustment except possibly after puberty, when emotional disturbance was more frequent and more serious. The height of the diabetic boys was less and the weight of the girls more than in the control group. Despite more frequent infections, antibody formation was intact. Special care was needed during these infections. That the diabetic child was absent from school more often than the non-diabetic child did not seem to affect scholastic standards.

The intelligence of diabetic children was measured by Ack and colleagues (1961). On the Stanford-Binet Form M those with an onset before the fifth birthday scored significantly below the controls. A relationship with hypoglycaemic attacks showed as a trend, but not significantly. The diabetic children with an onset after 5 years of age were no different from their siblings. In contrast, Etzwiler and Sines (1962) found 45 per cent of 74 juvenile diabetics with IQ above 110. Both Ack's team and those observers felt that educational difficulties existed and that as a group affected children were difficult to control. The former blamed the feeling of not being normal and of realizing the need for prolonged dependence.

Acceptance of the diagnosis and of limitations imposed by it is of the greatest importance. Among child health needs, adequate information and timely instruction in techniques of urine testing, diet control and insulin injection and regulation rank high. Almost all diabetic children are insulin dependent and need at least one and often two daily injections. All must exercise self-control over diet. As this involves sweets and cakes, which are 'reward' substances, success is difficult to achieve. Apart from these special needs, the child should be encouraged to lead as normal a life as possible. Because he is the best person to manage his own life, he must be taught to give his own injections, to recognize the symptoms of hypoglycaemia, to know how to correct it, and what to do to cope with inter-current infection and vomiting and before exercise. Every diabetic child should be sure of getting this help from someone.

Etzwiler (1962, 1967) in the USA, while recognizing the importance of this instruction, has stressed the difficulty of imparting to the child with diabetes a real understanding of the nature of his disease. He believes that attempts to make him look after his own diabetic treatment too early are harmful and that variation in readiness between individuals should be expected and the degree of readiness assessed. Three quarters of the 6- and 7-year-olds could interpret the urine test correctly and could recognize insulin reactions, but few could comprehend the significance of the blood sugar level or of acetone in the urine, or the difference between soluble and long acting insulins before the age of 12 years. A questionnaire on fundamentals was poorly answered by parents of diabetic children; and even a sample of general practitioners showed distinct evidence of ignorance. It would be of practical importance to make a similar survey in England and Wales.

With fewer than 9000 diabetic children in the community, most general practitioners will have no single diabetic child on his list. In the 53 practices (GPR) there were only 29 children under the age of 15 years consulting in the year, 10 of whom were at home. This limits experience of management and makes essential the availability of at least one physician, competent and knowledgeable, in each area. There is a strong case, too, for a specially trained health visitor to whom the diabetic child and his family can turn. Education at normal school is desirable, but adverse social circumstances or the absence of adequate mothering may lead to a need for foster care or residential nursery or school. Such special measures may be considered to be the only ways in which the child has a good chance of survival. Nevertheless, the aim is not merely to get the diabetic through childhood alive, but to ensure that in the process of growing up nothing is done to hamper his development physically, emotionally, intellectually and educationally. Perhaps the first of these requirements remains the most difficult to achieve, because knowledge is lacking about the way to prevent premature vascular damage. Retinopathy with increasing visual defect, nephropathy, cardiac and neurological lesions impair function and shorten life expectancy. Diabetic retinopathy is responsible for 13.1 per cent of all blindness in men and 18.2 per cent of all blindness in women at all ages (Sorsby 1972). Every step in management and treatment of the juvenile diabetic must be regarded in this context. The question of special diabetic clinic supervision is discussed below.

CYSTIC FIBROSIS (of the pancreas)

The basic defect in this complex disease escapes detection. That it is a genetically determined disease inherited as an autosomal recessive and that all exocrine glands are affected are established facts. Most of the babies are normal at birth. There is therefore a need to identify the baby with one of the basic defects and to prevent if possible the serious secondary results. These are malabsorption and nutritional failure from pancreatic disease, respiratory infection, once suspected but not proven to be aggravated by the presence of abnormal mucus, hepatic failure and portal hypertension, and sometimes sterility in the male due to blocked seminiferous tubules. In about 10 per cent, the newborn baby produces clinical evidence of acute intestinal obstruction from meconium ileus within the first week of life. Intestinal obstruction from impacted faeces may also occur later in childhood.

The availability of potent pancreatic preparations and the use of high protein diets should prevent under-nutrition. The real danger lies in progressive destruction of the lungs that results from repeated pulmonary infections, and it is the attempts to avoid such infections and to limit the damage caused by each attack that dominate the family's life.

Incidence at birth has been variously assessed, but 1 in 2500 live births in England and Wales provides a reasonably practical approximation.

This would introduce about 320 new children each year. If they all survived the maximum numbers in the population from birth to age 15 years at one time would be 4800. George and Norman (1971) have prepared life tables, based on 128 children, which show a considerable improvement in survival rates when the quinquennium 1964–68 is compared with the series 1943–64. The outlook appears better when the patients are entered in the series at birth rather than at the time of diagnosis. The worst outlook is for babies with meconium ileus entered at the time of diagnosis, with only 477 out of 1000 expected to survive to the fifth year. This compares with 956 survivors out of 1000 at 5 years of those without meconium ileus and entered at birth, of whom 704 would be expected to reach their sixteenth year. Since these tables were compiled, the surgical treatment of meconium ileus and general medical management have greatly improved the outlook. A study of 215 children attending a hospital between 1969 and 1973 shows that 79 per cent of those presenting with meconium ileus and 97 per cent of those not so presenting were alive at 5 years of age (Robinson and Norman 1975).

Translated into estimated numbers and assuming an annual entry of 320 new babies with cystic fibrosis, 45 are expected to be born with meconium ileus and 275 without it. The number of affected children requiring treatment during any one year would be about 3100. Continuing improvement in the effectiveness of treatment will increase life expectancy and the numbers of late survivors.

Diagnostic procedures

Direct measurement of pancreatic enzymes has not proved helpful. Attention is now mainly paid to the sodium or chloride contents of sweat, saliva or nail-clippings. Blood serum disturbs rhythmical ciliary movement in cultures of ciliated cells. While sometimes these tests yield unequivocal answers, there are unfortunate gray areas in which normal people, carriers of the gene and some affected patients overlap. There is as yet no technique for accurate fetal diagnosis. All doctors and nurses with responsibility for babies should be familiar with the earliest clinical symptoms.

Health needs

The siblings of known patients should always be screened for sodium or chloride content of sweat or saliva. No firm decision has yet been taken about the need to screen all newborn babies. Such special groups as babies being offered for adoption should certainly be screened as soon as there is a simple test giving a precise answer. A positive result should lead to a full discussion with prospective adopters of what is involved, but it is not necessarily an absolute contra-indication to adoption.

Another difficult problem is what therapeutic steps should be taken when the positive test is found in a baby who is clinically normal and when the question arises of 'prophylactic' antibiotics. The regulation of diet and the prescribing of pancreatic extracts is probably best begun in a hospital clinic and the routine supervision accepted as the responsibility of the general practitioner. Periodic visits to the paediatric clinic would be desirable through childhood. The most difficult part of management surrounds family action aimed at avoiding respiratory infection by methods which succeed only in producing over-anxiety and over-protection. The attainable objective is the prevention of lung damage when respiratory infections occur.

Turk (1964) quotes an American parent as saying 'no one can live a normal life if they have a cystic fibrosis child'. The questions that he was posing were these: Do the demands for and the cost of care for the cystic fibrosis child result in social and financial deprivation for all members of the family? Does the attention and energy required limit the parents' other activities or communication with the members of the family? There is little doubt that affirmative answers do often apply in England and Wales, but the cost of treatment is less of a financial burden than in the USA because drugs are provided free for children through the NHS. The cost of extra meat in the diet and of controlling the temperature in the bedroom together with the cost of wages lost and of travelling to hospital clinics without too great a risk of cross infection have still to be included in the family budget.

The cost in spare time and energy is measured in broken sleep, absence of family holidays and the need to give regular physiotherapy and postural drainage. To make matters worse, children may resist treatment at any age, but especially in adolescence. Mist tents are still in use and are still recommended, despite the lack of clear evidence of their value or of a well-founded theoretical basis for their use now that doubt exists about the abnormality of the mucus in the respiratory tract.

Perhaps of greater importance is the constant anxiety which is the enemy of happiness and the feeling that the family is being deprived of normal life. There are some special problems that defy perfect solutions. How can the child be protected sufficiently and at the same time develop independence? What restrictions are really needed to prevent respiratory infection? Should he go to school and risk infection or should he have a home tutor and lose the companionship and the social assets of school life? How can the other children in the family be helped to understand that it is the situation of the affected child that produces the demands and that they themselves are not being rejected?

The answers to these questions cannot be stereotyped. The severity of the case, the ability of parents to accept and adjust to their problems, the personality of the child, the condition of siblings must all influence decisions. That families all need counselling and that some need financial and housing help cannot be denied. The general practitioner and the medical social worker familiar with the special difficulties produced by the disease need the support of the hospital clinic. Here treatment and management plans can be reviewed by paediatricians, social workers and dietitians, with access to respiratory physiotherapy and to paediatric surgery for pulmonary and abdominal crises.

ADRENOGENITAL SYNDROME

This syndrome has profound effects on the lives of patient and family. A full discussion of intersex and pseudo-hermaphroditism would be out of place, but special reference is justified for a condition that does make great demands on a number of specialists spread over the whole of childhood. The syndrome results from a failure in the synthesis of cortisol and the defective enzyme is usually the 21 hydroxylase, although other enzymes have also been implicated. Attempts have been made at prenatal diagnosis through the measurement of steroids in amniotic fluid. The results are not sufficiently clear cut and inasmuch as urinary estimation in the newborn cannot always be interpreted accurately (Shackleton *et al.* 1972) much more work will have to be done before prenatal diagnosis becomes practicable. The advantage would be that virilization of the fetus might become preventable.

A more certain advantage would be the identification at birth of the salt-losing males. When the diagnosis is missed, surgical operations for example for suspected pyloric or intestinal obstruction can be fatal. The original regulation of steroid and metabolic treatment is best carried out in hospital. Careful biochemically controlled observation with attention to bodily growth is paralleled by parent counselling and the detailed explanation of the effects on sex life and of the possibilities offered by plastic surgery. The patient is naturally liable to be confused about sex identity.

The reported incidence varies from 1:5000 in parts of Switzerland (Prader) to 1:67 000 in Maryland (Childs). An accepted figure for England and Wales in 1:8000. This would mean, if correct, 100 new patients each year and if all survived there should be 1000 school children with adrenogenital syndrome. It is unlikely that so great a number is known in the school population. RGSR gives 13 deaths, 8 in the first year and HIPE 132 discharges and deaths from diseases of the adrenal glands (ICD 255). The 4 deaths in the first two weeks of life could have resulted from haemorrhage into the adrenal glands.

HAEMOPHILIA

Haemophilia is potentially a cause of chronic disability as well as creating in some patients heavy demands for emergency treatment. A sex-linked recessive inheritance is usual, but a family history is unknown in 30 per cent of patients. The Haemophilia Society estimates a total haemophilic population in the United Kingdom (not restricted to England and Wales) of between 2000 and 3000, of whom probably 1 in 10 have Christmas Disease. Half of them are expected to have enough of the deficient factor in their blood to be free from symptoms and in general not to need special treatment. The other half, classed as severe, require a great deal of medical and other services.

The true incidence of haemophilia is unknown, but estimates vary between 1 in 10 000 males (Netherlands) and 1 in 65 000 (Belgium). Accepted figures of prevalence for the United Kingdom lie between 1 in 13 000 and 1 in 20 000 total population. Applied to England and Wales an incidence of 1 in 10 000 males yields a figure of 40 new cases in 1971. Treatment at some stage will be needed for about 20 of them. Rizza from the Oxford Haemophilia Centre suggests the remarkably high incidence of 1 haemophilic to every 3000 or 4000 live male births, the severe form affecting 3 to 4 per 100 000 population. Using both the low and the high figures the total number of haemophilics in the school population in England and Wales could range from 600 to 2000 if all survived.

The main forms of haemophilia result from defects of factors VIII and IX. Classical haemophilia due to factor VIII deficiency has a prevalence of 60 to 70 per million population, Christmas disease (factor IX deficiency) of 8 to 10 and von Willebrand's disease of 10 to 20. All the other defects are rare accounting altogether for less than 5 per million of population (Biggs 1976).

A survey by the Haemophilia Society in 1967 of some 500 patients showed that 46 per cent were crippled. Three quarters (73.2 per cent) had become crippled before the age of 15 years and half of these (37.2 per cent of the total) before the age of 10 years. Undoubtedly, increased survival will increase prevalence; on the other hand, modern treatment, if fully available and fully used, must reduce the amount of physical disability.

Haemophilics 'need to take their place in society as well-integrated, independent individuals, able to earn a salary and support their families' (Britten *et al.* 1966). Some authorities favour special schools for haemophilics although this takes them out of their place in children's society. Out of 322 of school age no less than 150 either had home tuition or were missing more than a quarter of school time. Much depends on the frequency of bleeding episodes. School masters should be encouraged to take into normal schools the mildly and many of the moderately affected children. For the severely affected the benefits of immediately available treatment may outweigh the disadvantages of separation from parents and home. Emergency treatment by parents at home is becoming available and should reduce both the permanent joint damage and the need for special residential schools.

Bronks and Blackburn (1968) in Sheffield conducted a follow-up study of 135 known haemophilics and found 65 per cent working. In 37 there was thought to be emotional disturbance, in 41 none and in the remaining 57 there was doubt. The age range was wide (one of them over 65 years old) so that the older patients were probably less severely affected, since the less well organized treatment of earlier times would not have been adequate for survival of severely affected haemophilics. This is shown when the proportions of haemophilics in the different age groups are compared with the proportions of normal children in the general population. In a population of haemophilics, children under 15 years formed 32.6 per cent compared with the normal 23 per cent. The proportion of 15- to 24-year-old haemophilics was twice that of the general population and the age group 45 years and over comprised only 9.6 per cent compared with 37.6 per cent.

Health needs

Haemophilic treatment, both emergency, and therefore on a 24-hour basis, and supervisory, is provided in 36 designated centres in England and Wales of which 13 are in London. Staffing shortages exist and the wide areas for which some centres are responsible limit the effectiveness of treatment. Expertise cannot operate if essential supplies of concentrates of factor VIII and IX, especially of cryoprecipitate, are lacking and this involves Fractionation Centres and Blood Banks. Early treatment, which is of the greatest importance in prevention of crippling, is only possible for families who have accepted the realities of their situation and have adjusted to them. The unco-operative family has an urgent need for psycho-paediatrics in the interests of the child. Dental attention forms one important part of supervision. The prevalence of haemophilia could be reduced, but, on account of the frequency of mutation, not eliminated, by preventing the live birth of all males in families known to be affected. Such an extreme measure does not recommend itself to the Working Party.

MUSCULAR DYSTROPHY

The incidence of muscular dystrophy has been estimated as about 30 per 100 000 live births (Dubowitz 1973). This would produce some 240 affected children for every annual cohort. No-one knows the exact prevalence, but assuming that the condition is diagnosed by the age of 5 years and the majority of affected children survive to reach their fifteenth birthday, there would be 2400 in the school population, a prevalence rate of 3.2 per 10 000. Of the six types only Duchenne pseudohypertrophic muscular dystrophy is numerically important during school life. Limb-girdle and facio-scapulo-humeral types begin in the second decade; distal, ocular, and congenital types, such as central core disease and glycogenosis are fortunately rare. This is not to say that their medical needs may be ignored. They are included in the small numbers of unclassified orthopaedic conditions requiring help with locomotion.

The Duchenne type begins to show at about 3 years of age. Diagnostic examination includes enzyme tests for child and parents and for the child possibly muscle biopsy and electro-myography. Early examination is needed, especially for the younger male siblings of affected boys. Genetic counselling and amniocentesis for fetal sexing should be available. Child and parents require much morale support while anxiety and muscular weakness increase. Sooner or later and usually by the age of 10 years the child is almost completely or completely chairbound, with the need for a hand and later an electrically operated chair.

From time to time claims are made for treatments which up to now have never been confirmed. Hospital admission is likely for trial of such treatments, as they continue to be proposed.

Normal or physically handicapped school is usually possible for a few years after the chairbound stage has been reached. With some families continued care at home presents too many problems, so that admission to a residential school is necessary. Attempts are made at this stage to prevent the development of fixed deformities of the lower limbs and spine. As with general treatment, so with this special preventive treatment, recommended methods have proved disappointing. The end result of wasting and fixed deformities of feet and ankles, knees, hips and spine require all the emotional resources of the child and his family. There is, besides, the physical strain of manhandling the older patient. Neither physiotherapy nor orthopaedic surgery have proved effective in the long term.

The clinical impression that affected boys are educationally retarded has been substantiated by many recent reviews. Dubowitz (1965) found among 27 boys with the Duchenne type that half came into the mildly mentally handicapped group while one in ten was severely mentally handicapped, one in seven was in the low normal range and only one in nine above the average. He observed deterioration with age in a limited prospective study suggesting that the disease process might affect the central nervous system as well as the voluntary muscles and the heart. There is also the possibility that apathy engendered by a knowledge of failing power and hopeless prognosis may contribute to the deterioration. Were it possible to inject an element of hope into the home or the school environment, some of this deterioration might prove to be preventable. On the other hand a dulling of awareness could be regarded as a blessing in disguise.

Clinical interest in the associated cardiomyopathy and in the decreasing vital capacity, as the thoracic cage becomes increasingly deformed, has not, so far, been matched by any therapeutic advance. Death during the later years of the second decade is usually associated with acute respiratory infection. The annual number of these deaths is not identifiable in RGSR. There were 72 deaths, 23 in the first year and 20 between 10 and 15 in 1971 in the hereditary and familial neuromuscular disorders (ICD 330–333). HIPE estimates 365 discharges and deaths.

A more hopeful prognosis for survival is possible in the autosomal, rather than in the sex-linked recessive type of Duchenne dystrophy and also in the rarer types of dystrophy mentioned above. Muscle weakness develops more slowly between non-progressive periods. All the problems of chronic physical handicap arise, acceptance, adjustment to the imposed limitation on life and career, and a need for all the morale support that can be mobilized.

The 53 practices (GPR) record 33 childhood consultations during the year for the 'other diseases of the central nervous system' which includes the hereditary and familial. The general practitioner is likely to meet affected children seldom. His contribution is to pick up the early evidence of failing motor ability and to maintain a medical interest and to strengthen flagging spirits while the affected child remains in his family's care at home. Practical difficulties arise over the child's comfort as fixed deformities, especially those of the spine, develop, and over the prescription of antibiotics in the presence of respiratory tract infections. A watching brief over electric chairs or other prosthesis can be of great help. Also to be watched is the effect of the downward course of the child on the younger male siblings.

MALIGNANT NEOPLASMS

Paediatric oncology has become a more important subject with the multiplication of methods of attack on cancer cells. Refinements of radiotherapy and chemotherapy, together with a wider use of surgery for metastases have produced an atmosphere of hope. Table 17.1 is not designed to dampen optimism, although its message is that, except for retinoblastoma, neuroblastoma and Hodgkin's disease, the annual deaths remain too near the level of the new registrations.

The Standing sub-committee on Cancer of the Central Health Services Council (Cancer 1971) estimates the yearly number of new cases of malignant disease likely to be encountered in a population of two million as 6056. This would include 47 children under the age of 15 years, giving an expected total of 1150 for 1971. This group, amounting

Table 17.1. Malignant neoplasms in England and Wales 1971
Number of deaths and of patients newly registered. 1–14 years

		Newly registered (*Taylor* 1972)	*Deaths* (*RGSR*)
ICD			
170	Bone	45	27
189–0	Kidney		
	Wilms tumor	70	44
190	Eye		
	retinoblastoma	25	5
191–2	Brain and CNS		
	neuroblastoma	265	210
200	Lymphosarcoma	80	42
210	Hodgkin's disease	40	15
204–7	Leukaemia		
	all forms	300	339
		825	682
	Remainder		80
	aged 0–4 years		277
	,, 5–9 ,,		287
	,, 10–14 ,,		198
140–209	All malignant neoplasms		Total 762

to only 0.77 per cent is likely to become lost among 147 000 adult cancer patients. And there is a second message from the table. Nearly half of the deaths from malignant disease occur in the younger age group (0–4 years) and only a quarter of them in the older (10–14). The latter are mainly tumours of brain, which are fairly evenly spread, and of bone which are concentrated in the older age group.

The rare sites for malignant tumours, such as the liver, bladder, testis and ovaries, and the majority of patients with retinoblastoma and Wilms tumour present in the first and second years of life.* All of these facts and figures, while strongly supporting the proposals for oncological centres, suggest that paediatric oncology should be a function of special paediatric centres rather than a minute fraction of the work of general adult centres. There should, of course, be close co-operation between the two, especially over basic and therapeutic research.

The need for paediatric nursing care in hospital, for separate paediatric out-patient attendance for the inevitable periodic follow up consultations, together with the need for radiographers and haematology technicians experienced in the handling of the very young patient, provide formidable arguments for special paediatric centres. There is, too, the humane consideration of parent counselling. The realization that a baby or child, always and properly regarded as healthy, has malignant disease strikes parents especially hard. Confirmation of diagnosis is followed by attempts at treatment of varying severity. Death can usually be postponed, even when it is not prevented, so that the parents face long months of uncertainty when hope alternates with despair. Management is likely to be conducted in a more satisfactory manner by a team with special experience of family care.

The needs of management and treatment could logically be provided in four oncology centres for England and Wales. In such centres all sufferers could receive the best available treatment and expertise could grow, especially if treatment protocols were agreed on a country-wide or better still an international basis. The disadvantages are that many of the children would be far from home when in hospital and journeys for follow up examinations would be long and costly. The suggestion that local specialists cannot retain clinical charge of their patients is likely to be resented. At present the work of the Northern and Southern Advisory Committees and of the special MRC Committee on the treatment of

*Routine surveillance of infants from 6 to 24 months should include a careful palpation of the abdomen for evidence of enlargement of a kidney. Those patients fortunate enough to be diagnosed before the second birthday have a much better chance of survival.

solid tumours in childhood should be encouraged. The attempts to secure some standardization of diagnostic and therapeutic measures should allow the essential comparison of results on which and only on which can improvements in treatment be obtained. It is to be hoped that this co-operation will lead in the end to a local demand for the establishment of paediatric oncology centres where the whole management and treatment may be conducted in a paediatric atmosphere where humanity rubs shoulders with research.

CHAPTER 18

Certain metabolic disorders and variants

Modern laboratory methods have led to the discovery of a number of enzyme deficiencies and variations in metabolic pathways. Apart from providing a scientific basis for the understanding of the nature of some genetically determined diseases, the discoveries have led to treatment, of both curative and preventive kinds. The actual numbers of affected families are small, but because of the demands for large-scale administrative, supervisory and therapeutic measures their importance is not to be measured by their prevalence. Screening programmes are required for early diagnosis, dietary treatment is costly and needs careful medical supervision and termination of pregnancy may be advised. As a 'growing point' in medicine also the subject earns a place in any paediatric training scheme. For these reasons what may seem a surprisingly large space is allotted here to complement the introductory statements in the chapter on the newborn (Chapter 3).

Some account follows of galactosaemia, phenylketonuria, cystinosis, Hartnup 'disease', maple syrup urine disease, histidinaemia, homocystinuria, cystinuria and the hyperaminoacidurias.

GALACTOSAEMIA

Urinary screening of newborn babies by the Guthrie test or by the fluorescence test of Beutler and Baluda (1966) reveals the presence of galactosuria. A birth incidence as high as 1 in 35 000 has been demonstrated in New York, but the Council of Europe's Working Party gives only 1 in 61 000, and the figure from the 'world literature' of screening is 1 : 75 000. In classical form the complete absence in homozygotes of the enzyme, galactose-1-phosphate uridyl transferase, causes clinical symptoms within the first 5 to 7 days of life or earlier. Unfortunately for accurate quantification past surveys did not recognize all the variants (Beutler *et al*. 1965).

In deficiencies of such absolute rarity producing numbers of the order of 20 fresh examples each year or only 13 if the 1 : 61 000 estimate be accepted, the presence of a fertile pair of married heterozygotes in any population studied must seriously influence the figures. Too often predictions of incidence are based on the discovery of 2 or 3 affected babies in the total group tested, on relating the numbers of identified babies to the total number of known but untested births in the area in which the laboratory is sited, or on expectations derived from an estimate of gene frequencies. The cost of screening programmes in manpower, laboratory space as well as in money should only be measured against an accurately established birth incidence. On the other hand, although absolutely rare, classical galactosaemia is one cause of preventable death, or if the baby lives, of preventable severe mental handicap. An early clinical diagnosis is usually possible and is sufficient for satisfactory preventive treatment. All child health personnel should be aware of the presenting symptoms and signs. The urine of all sick newborn babies should be tested for galactose.

The *health needs* include the prescription and regular supervision of the diet. The use of prepared foods makes periodic review of all that contain carbohydrate essential. The informed general practitioner should be able to provide routine supervision and to prescribe special low lactose milk. A metabolic unit in the main area children's hospital is justified by the importance of the treatment in preventing damage to body, eyes and intelligence. If there be as many as 20 fresh cases each year and if all survive, there should be about 300 affected children at any one time in England and Wales.

PHENYLKETONURIA

Phenylpyruvic oligophrenia was the first of the enzymopathies to attract attention as a possibly preventable form of severe mental handicap. Neonatal screening, dietary treatment and clinic supervision are already accepted as essential in the National Health Service. Evidence is gathering of the beneficial effect of diet despite many earlier difficulties and unforeseen complications. The Guthrie test is still used predominantly. The diagnosis must never rest on the screening test but depends on studies of blood and urine. Chromatographic measurement of phenylalanine levels in the blood are required for accurate estimates of prevalence. In their absence figures may well vary from one area to another and babies who are not truly in danger of tissue damage may be submitted unnecessarily to a form of dietary control that is costly and not without risk. The critical factors are a dangerous level of phenylalanine variously stated to be 30, above 20 and above 15 mg per 100 ml and persistence of hyperphenylalaninaemia. A transient excess is encountered.

Variants, termed atypical PKU, with some degree of persistent hyperphenylalaninaemia but of normal mentality have been found in screened populations, the reported incidence varying between 1:11 000 and 1:200 000.*

The risks of treatment are failure to thrive and even brain damage when the blood phenylalanine level is too low (it should be kept between 3 and 7 mg per 100 ml) and the emotional problems to which all children are liable who need strictly controlled diets for long periods. When successfully treated females become pregnant, a high phenylalanine level becomes dangerous since by crossing the placenta it could damage the fetus.

The Council of Europe's Working Party summarizing population studies in eight European countries estimated an incidence of 1 in 8000 newborn. In 1969, using Komrower's figure, about 118 newborn babies should have been affected. The maximum numbers in the child population if every one survived to 15 years would be 1770 in England and Wales. The USA figure based on nearly 8 million newborns is 1:14 000. The birth incidence varies between different ethnic groups.

CYSTINOSIS

The infantile form of cystine storage disease like the benign adult (type II) form and the intermediate adolescent (type III) form is transmitted by an autosomal recessive gene. The three forms may depend on abnormalities in different gene loci. The basic defect locks cystine within the lysosomes; its exact nature is not known. The affected baby appears normal at birth and makes normal progress for a time. Growth slows down as appetite is lost and vomiting and constipation combine with polyuria, polydipsia and high fever. The clinical picture on which diagnosis depends is of de Toni-Debré-Fanconi's syndrome with rickets, vitamin D resistance, hypophosphataemia, acidosis, glycosuria and a general aminoaciduria. Aminoaciduria may be present in some affected neonates or in the early weeks of life. Cystinosis affects, besides bone growth, the retina and the cornea producing marked photophobia, and reduced pigmentation of the hair. The most serious result is nephro-

*To avoid continuing unnecessary dietary treatment, the MRC Committee on Phenylketonuria recommends confirmatory tests at 4 and 9 months. Atypical phenylketonuria is likely to be diagnosed in those babies whose blood phenylalanine levels did not exceed 20 mg per 100 ml. There is as yet no certainty about the length of time of dietary treatment for the classical condition.

pathy, a combined glomerular and tubular damage with a characteristic swan-neck appearance of the proximal tubule. Death from uraemia occurs within the first decade, a circumstance that raises the question of renal replacement. The benign 'adult' form has been reported in children (Brubaker *et al.* 1970). The adolescent form includes rickets and nephropathy without retinal or pigmentary changes. These forms are not lethal despite cystine storage. Diagnosis depends on finding a general aminoaciduria and cystine crystals in the tissues. Crystal profiles have been seen on electron microscopy of material from renal biopsy and bone marrow before crystals could be seen by slit lamp examination of the cornea (Witzleben *et al.* 1972).

Prevalence

Levy in the Massachusetts neonatal survey found 21 cases giving an incidence at birth of 1 in 16 000; this would produce 50 new babies each year, if applicable in England and Wales. Heterozygotes have excessive cystine in cultured fibroblasts and in polymorphs and monocytes. Various attempts at treatment have been made. To identify the whole group in the childhood population and for the time being to keep careful records will prepare the way for rational treatment. This is likely to be delayed until the presumed enzyme defect has been found. Low cystine and methionine diets and penicillamine have not proved satisfactory. Dithiothreitol reduces the cystine in tissues *in vitro* and has been given intravenously to patients (Goldman *et al.* 1970). None of this is practicable at present, but should a screening programme become available the problem of supervision and advice for heterozygous parents will need to be faced.

HARTNUP 'DISEASE'

Although the Hartnup family contained children with a photosensitive skin rash, neurological signs and hyperaminoaciduria, the existence of a disease entity has not been confirmed. The aminoaciduria is due to a defect in amino-acid transport, which does not always produce symptoms. It is inherited as an autosomal recessive character. The defect, existing in both intestinal and renal tubule, involves tryptophan and phenylalanine always and to some extent methionine, lysine and glycine (Shih *et al.* 1971). The massive urinary excretion of all neutral amino acids except proline and hydroxyproline produces a characteristic chromatographic pattern. Plasma tryptophan is reduced. Large doses of nicotinamide are recommended but do not reduce the aminoaciduria.

Surveys of mentally handicapped children have shown that defective tryptophan transport is not always associated with ataxia or skin lesions.

Hartnup 'disease' was not included in the Council of Europe study. Levy and his colleagues in the Massachusetts survey found 18 patients with a birth incidence of 1 in 18 000. Each year the birth of 44 Hartnup babies may be expected in England and Wales, and since this is certainly not a lethal defect, there should be 660 children with defective tryptophan transport in the child population at any one time. To what extent health is jeopardized is uncertain.

MAPLE SYRUP URINE DISEASE

MSUD is given an incidence of 1 in 81 091 by the Council of Europe Working Party on the basis of 9 patients, all but one identified by the Guthrie test for leucin and none found up to 1971 in Great Britain. Levy identified 5 newborns out of some 840 000, an incidence of 1 : 170 000. The most recent 'world literature' incidence is 1 : 220 000. Neurological disturbance, failure of development and the characteristic urine smell are usually noticed in the early days of life. Three branched-chain amino-acids, valine, leucine and isoleucine are found in high concentration in the urine. Death occurs within the first few months. The earliest possible diagnosis and dietary treatment hold out some hope.

HISTIDINAEMIA

This is one of the variants about the pathogenicity of which uncertainty persists. Symptoms attributed to histidinaemia develop slowly and include delayed speech and retardation of both physical and mental growth and development. Thalhammer (1970) using the Guthrie test found 3 patients in studying a population of 36 462, a neonatal incidence of 1 in 12 000. There were 62 false positives. Levy *et al.* (1971) demonstrated delay in the maturation of histidine transaminase in the neonatal period. Transient histidinaemia with histidinuria is expected in any newborn screening programme in 20 newborns for every patient with the hereditary defect of histidase. The Council of Europe found a prevalence of 1 in 19 972 and Levy in Massachusetts of 1 in 18 000. But it remains uncertain whether excess of histidine damages the tissues and no absolute relationship has been established with mental defect. A mother with histidinaemia has given birth to a child with no evidence of disease or deficiency by the age of $4\frac{1}{2}$ years (Neville *et al.* 1971). A low histidine diet is available and in use, but at present in USA babies identified through screening are being left untreated.

HOMOCYSTINURIA

Homocystinuria, diagnosed through the Guthrie test for methionine or urine chromatography, is given an incidence of 1 in 185 145 by the Council of Europe through the positive screening of six patients. Although 100 cases were reported from 1962–68, the incidence from the 'world literature' on screening is 1 : 220 000. Three forms have been described. In the classical form the baby is normal at birth, but growth and development become abnormal as the result of cystathione synthetase deficiency which interrupts the metabolic pathway from methionine to cystine. The enzyme is normally found in liver, brain and cultured fibroblasts. Its deficiency causes elevation of homocystine and methionine in blood and urine. The extremities are long, muscle tone is poor and one third of the children share many features with Marfan's syndrome including dislocation of the lens of the eye. The combination of osteoporosis, which occurs in 35 per cent, with Marfan's syndrome is especially damaging to the spine and thorax. Intellectual deterioration is noted in 77 per cent (Beals 1969) and seizures are commonly present. 'Stickiness' of platelets possibly caused by high serum homocystine levels results in diffuse thrombo-embolic incidents. The two other types are due respectively to a defect in vitamin B12 and in folate metabolism. The clinical picture can be less severe than in the classical form. Carson who was an early investigator has shown that treatment with pyridoxine returns the biochemical abnormalities to normal, although not in all patients. Wilcken and Turner (1973) have found a similar biochemical improvement, enhanced by the administration of folic acid. The case for screening for homocystinuria, despite the expectation of finding only five or six affected newborns each year, is strengthened by these encouraging results.

CYSTINURIA

This results from defective renal tubular and intestinal mucosal transport. Cysteine, lysine, ornithine and arginine are excreted in the urine in increased amounts and renal calculi may form. The serious results are pain, progressive loss of renal function and the need for surgical treatment. Blood amino-acid levels remain normal and the urine has to be screened. Reported incidence in newborn screening studies vary between 1 in 2000 and 1 in 15 000 and it is certain that several distinct genetic groups exist. The prevention of urinary calculi due to cystinuria is being attempted, the methods suggested being high water intake, alkalinization of the urine, d-penicillamine and a low methionine diet. The prevalence of renal calculi in childhood is low, but preventive measures probably should be taken early in life.

HYPER-AMINOACIDURIAS

Large-scale screening programmes carried out in many populations inevitably reveal peculiarities. At the same time elaborate investigation of non-thriving infants, especially with defects in the central nervous system, has demonstrated associations with excretion of excessive amounts of amino-acids singly or in combination. Delay in maturation either of specific enzymes or excretory pathways leads to transient amino-acidurias. Quantification is for these reasons an unreliable business and it must suffice here to refer only to a few tentative conclusions.

Transient rises in blood levels of tyrosine (up to 8 mg per 100 ml) have been found in as many as 3 per cent of neonatal populations. While persistently high levels are found in liver disease and as a genetic abnormality in some families in association with rickets, hepatic cirrhosis and glycosuria, the question has been raised of a harmful effect of transient tyrosinaemia on ultimate intellectual performance in some large premature babies (Menkes *et al.* 1971).

Hyperglycinaemia is found in some children with recurrent ketotic attacks and a dangerous ammonia intoxication in a few children with arginino-succinic aciduria. Defective iminoglycine transport and high levels of lysine and ornithine have also been noted. The whole question of blood and urine screening, its timing, its importance, its place in preventive medicine needs to be kept under periodic review in relation to programmes of Child Health.

SCREENING FOR CERTAIN BLOOD DISORDERS

Glucose-6-phosphate dehydrogenase (G-6-PD) deficiency

Deficiency of G-6-PD function in RBC can be demonstrated by the fluorescent test of Beutler. The defect is not so much a suppression of the enzyme as the formation of one or other functionally inadequate mutants. A few families of undoubtedly pure English stock have been shown to carry the gene, but among African blacks the incidence may be higher than 10 per cent. The enzymatic activity of the African mutant is about 10 per cent of normal in comparison with the zero activity in Mediterranean peoples (Arab, Greek, Italian and Sephardic Jews). In the immigrant black African population, the results of exposure to the agents that provoke haemolysis should not be the most severe. Apart from fava beans, the cause of Baghdad Spring Fever, drugs derived from quinoline, certain sulfa drugs, especially furadantin, acetyl-salicylic acid and PAS are the most likely to cause a haemolytic crisis. Avoidance of these and other known provocative agents in a susceptible population should make screening unnecessary.

Sickle cell haemoglobin

This variant of haemoglobin A is found, almost exclusively, in black Africans, but for the first few months of life in only small amounts. The importance of screening is in the identification of heterozygotes who carry the trait and the distinction between heterozygotes and homozygotes may be difficult before the age of 6 months. The blood of the homozygote contains some 90 per cent haemoglobin S and such children require supervision usually under hospital care for any prophylactic and crisis treatment that is available. The heterozygotes with 35 to 50 per cent haemoglobin S remain healthy unless especially stressed or exposed to extremely low oxygen tension atmospheres. The most cogent reason for their identification is for genetic counselling. While screening during the period 6 months to 18 months could protect them from developing symptoms, the important time is before marriage and the production of children. The positive screening may be forgotten if it has occurred in infancy. The risk to children of the union of two heterozygotes should be known before procreation in the susceptible population. In a family at risk the paediatrician, the general practitioner or the school medical officer should take responsibility for preparing the growing children with accurate information about what may lie ahead. Huntsman and Lehmann (1974) stress the need for good personal, family and community hygiene, the prompt treatment of infection, the maintenance of hydration and avoidance of exposure to cold besides regular doses of folic acid.

Disorders of sphingolipid metabolism

The growth of more exact knowledge about lipid metabolism has led to the identification of a number of deficiencies in enzyme systems, including lysosomal enzymes. Unfortunately as yet there has been little therapeutic advance. Most of the disorders are inherited as autosomal recessives. Materials are deposited in the central nervous system which cause progressive mental deterioration, sensory loss, including loss of vision, seizures, generalized spasticity and death in the early years of life. In the absence of effective treatment, the present approach is towards fetal diagnosis as a prelude to termination of pregnancy. The prevalence of these forms of storage disease remains unknown, but the commonest are the infantile form of amaurotic idiocy (classical Tay-Sachs disease), Gaucher's and Niemann-Pick's diseases and metachromatic leukodystrophy.

Tay-Sachs disease (GM_2 gangliosidosis) has been the most intensively studied. The defective enzyme, hexosaminidase A, can be measured in cultivated fibroblasts (Nadler *et al.* 1970) from amniotic fluid at 13 weeks, leaving sufficient time for termination. More recently (Friedland *et al.* 1971) claims have been made for successful diagnosis by studies of amniotic fluid, although only in the classical and not in the rare variant forms. Heterozygotes and homozygotes may also be discovered by serum hexosaminidase assay (O'Brien *et al.* 1970). There is no special population at risk for variants of abnormal sphingolipid metabolic defects, but Tay-Sachs disease in its classical form is found largely but not exclusively among Jews. Facilities should, therefore, exist for selective population studies and for families who have already produced an affected offspring. That fetal diagnosis of most of these enzyme defects will be practicable is a reasonable expectation. The size of the problem should be definable within a few years. Meanwhile appropriate laboratory techniques should be provided in centres where enzyme defects are investigated.

When the diagnosis results from clinical examinations during infancy or early childhood, the parents have to face the prospect of a steady deterioration. The final stages are hard to bear and residential hospital placement may be necessary. The fact that the affected child is likely to die, while bringing a solution to the problem, accentuates both guilt feelings about bringing the child into the world with abnormal genes inherited from them and fears about the outcome of future pregnancies.

Health needs. The major health need in children affected by inborn errors of metabolism (hereditary metabolic diseases) is acceptance by the family that the diagnosis and prognosis are correct. Only then can they face the absolute need for the prolonged and accurate control of diet when this is available. Without family co-operation and without the confidence of the child as he grows through all the emotionally troubled early years with the feeling of 'being different', the enterprise will fail. The needs in personnel and in dietary regulation can best be met by doctors working in clinics where everything is geared to the happiness, the comfort and convenience of the family during the repeated and sometimes lengthy visits. The clinic staff must include, besides the doctor and the social worker, the dietitian, the laboratory technicians and access to the educational psychologist. Because the efficiency of treatment in many of the conditions is not finally established, careful and, if possible, standardized records should be kept, and bodily and intellectual growth and emotional adjustment periodically reviewed. Liaison between the centres should be close with regular meetings recognized as an integral part of the work, and results should be pooled. No doctor in isolation should take responsibility for the long term care and supervision of the one patient whom he happens to diagnose.

Reference is made in the chapter on mental health to the possibility of preventing damage to intelligence resulting from inherited metabolic errors. Obviously success depends on population screening. In some areas screening is established, but the question remains open whether the cost in man-power, laboratory space and equipment and in money justifies the adoption of screening techniques for the whole population. Komrower (1976) and his colleagues in Manchester estimate the present screening cost per baby fully tested and including the sophisticated tests for doubtful positives as 24 pence. The further testing of those with postive screening tests falls naturally into the routine work of the laboratory. In 1971 a complete population screening of all live born babies would have cost about £188 000. A rough estimate taking the highest claimed birth incidence figures, would be of 500 new patients each year.*

To neglect prophylactic methods of proven success because of capital outlay and high running costs in a National Health Service cannot be ethically defended. Nevertheless, doubts still remain both about the interpretation of tests and the absolute effectiveness of treatment. Centres already established should be encouraged to extend their work. Certain absolute essentials are that defined and circumscribed total populations should be studied and that records should be kept with meticulous care. Supervisory clinics must be organized where dietary advice and appropriate drug treatment can be provided on patterns standardized as much as possible. Close links are also essential with obstetric departments to regulate amniocentesis and pregnancy termination, and with psychiatric and social welfare departments. More is at stake than the physical and

*The Massachusetts team (Levy *et al.* 1972) reckon that each urine screening test costs one dollar, which would be equivalent to an annual expenditure of £352 000 for the population of England and Wales (100 per cent tested and 6 per cent retested).

mental health of the babies and children. The future well-being of the family caught up in these problems matters much more from the point of view of the community as a whole. Genetic counselling for the individual families and epidemiological studies should be included in any scheme from the results of which it is intended that guide lines for the future should be drawn.

An argument frequently employed to support the expense of screening is the high cost of care for a mentally handicapped patient, for example after the brain damage from phenylalanine which is assumed to be preventable. The validity of this comparison of costs is extremely doubtful and serves only to draw attention away from the basic lack of knowledge of answers to many vital questions. Among them, given that the population is provided with screening tests and the recommended dietary control, does the number of children with phenylpyruvic oligophrenia diminish? When this has been established as true and when and if the other enzymopathies are shown to be identifiable by screening and the damage which they do to be preventable by treatment, a total programme for the whole country must be provided. Much social welfare support is needed by families whose health, happiness and even stability of marriage is often stressed by what they feel about and by what they have to do for an affected child.

Any discussion of screening programmes would be incomplete without mention of social attitudes. Ideally laboratory services should be available for all. While for research purposes 'whole' populations without exception are highly desirable if not essential, the introduction of statutory screening would be not only an undesirable infringement of personal and parental liberty of choice but would also grant a right of screening to all. Little time would elapse before claims for compensation would arise, with all their inevitable legal and ethical complications. Parents, patients and doctors must always preserve the right to opt out.

Table 18.1. Incidence on screening for certain metabolic variants

		WHO	*CE*	*K* n=169 400	*Mass* n=*variable*	*Expected new* 1971 n=783 155 *max*	*min*
N	*Phenylketonuria*	1:10 000	1:8000 (544)	1:6776 (25)	1:15 000 (66:1 012 017)	115	52
	'Atypical' Phenylketonuria			1:85 000 (2)	1:17 000 (60:1 012 017)	46	9
	Cystinuria (complete)				1:15 000 (23:350 176)		52
	Hartnup 'disease'				1:16 000 (22:350 176)		49
N	*Histidinaemia*		1:12 000 (18)	1:24 200 (7)	1:18 000 (20:350 176)	66	32
	Hyperprolinaemia			1:84 700 (2)			9
NF	*Galactosaemia*	1:25 000	1:61 000 (11)		1:120 000 (5:588 827)	31	7
N	*Maple Syrup Urine Disease MSUD*		1:81 000 (9)		1:176 000 (5:872 660)	10	4
	Fructosuria						
N	*Homocystinuria*		1:185 000 (6)	1:169 400 (1)	1:160 000 (3:480 271)	5	4
N	*Tyrosinaemia (hereditary)*		1:385 000 (1)				2
?F	*Cystic fibrosis of pancreas*	1:1500 1:8000				522	97 (320)
?F	*Adrenogenital syndrome*	1:67 000 1:5000				156	11
	Pseudo-cholinesterase deficiency						
	Wilson's disease	1:100 000				8	
	Hereditary immune deficiences	1:100 000				8	
N	glucose-6-phosphate-dehydrogenase-deficiency						
7/12	Haemoglobinopathy						
F	Tay-Sachs disease.						

N=neonatal screening; F=fetal screening; figures ( ) actual numbers in a study; titles in italic indicate reasonably satisfactory treatment.
WHO – Technical Report 401 (1968)
CE – Council of Europe Mass Screening . . . hereditary enzymopathies, Strasbourg 1972
K – GM Komrower *Ann. clin. Biochem.*, (1972) **9**, 126
Mass – Massachusetts metabolic disorders screening program. H. L. Levy *et al.*, *Pediat.* (1972) **49**, 825

Table 18.2. Hereditary enzymopathies and proteinopathies which may produce clinical consequences and for which screening and/or treatment are possible
(Based on Council of Europe Working Party 1972)

1	Glactosaemia
2	Phenlyketonuria
3	Cystinosis
4	Hartnup 'disease'
5	Histidinaemia
6	Homocystinuria
7	Maple syrup urine disease
8	Cystic fibrosis (of the pancreas)
9	Adrenogenital syndrome
10	Sphingolipidoses
11	Hereditary immune deficiencies
12	G-6-PD deficiency
13	Fructose intolerance
14	Tyrosinosis
15	Cystinuria
16	Lesch-Nyhan disease
17	Glycogenosis
18	Thyroxin synthesis disorders
19	Wilson's disease
20	Vitamin D resistant rickets
21	Pitressin resistant diabetes insipidus
22	Haemoglobinopathy S
23	Thalassaemia

Levy lists other aminoacidurias for example iminoglycinuria, argininosuccinic aciduria, cystathioninuria, and some hyperaminoacidaemia such as phenylalanine, glycine, lysine and ornithine.

CHAPTER 19

*Accidents and injuries**

The changing pattern of disease in childhood has increased the relative importance of accidents and injuries. This is not yet reflected either in training or in practice. The dictionary concept of 'an event without an apparent cause' has become less acceptable since some apparent causes have been revealed by placing accidents in the context of family and social life and applying to causation the techniques of clinical research and of epidemiology. While chance plays its part in that, for example, the child must be near the boiling water before it can be scalded, there are epidemiological patterns of risk for certain accidents both as regards peak-age incidence and sex distribution. Douglas (1958) has drawn attention to the influence of birth date on burns which have a peak incidence in the second year of life. Children born in autumn and winter are in greater danger from fires and heating apparatus when they make their first faltering attempts to walk. Boys are in general more liable to accident than girls.

The Newcastle team was led to classify accidents along with alimentary infections, retarded growth and squints, as diseases of the social environment, noting especially the importance of bad housing and poor quality maternal care. In Douglas's study, although more infants in the lower income groups had burns and scalds in the first year of life, a correlation of accidents after the first year with housing conditions was not found. Accidents affected 29 per cent of children in the best housing and 30 per cent in the worst. Furthermore, the children who had accidents were bigger and stronger, and fewer had defects of sight, hearing, heart or lungs or poor ratings for alertness. The mothers were more prone to worry, the children appeared to be the more adventurous, but, as most observers have found, maternal care was less good.

Recent studies have drawn attention to behavioural and psychological factors. Husband and Hinton (1972) have described children with repeated accidents as of extrovert personality often with associated family problems, including organic disease and psychological illness. The implication of this work is that when children have repeated accidents, however mild their character, binding the wound is not enough. 'Accidental injury

*Tables relating to this chapter from HIPE and RGSR will be found in Appendices VI, VII, VIII, IX

ceases to be fortuitous, but becomes an event whose understanding must accompany efforts to help the injured child and his family' (Martin 1970). If this be the truth, the casualty department must increase its awareness of the need for social work and for psychological insight.

The social and psychological elements in child abuse are well recognized. What is not certain is the number of injuries, particularly during the first two years, which should arouse the suspicion of abuse. Jackson (1972), reviewing one hundred child casualties in a hospital well alerted to the possibility of abuse, has found 18 where abuse had not been considered, but which showed, on further study, the highly suspicious features of delayed presentation and inconsistent history. The doctor regards the cause of an accident as clear when a credible account of the happening can be given. Newer thinking, that the injury is often a clue to some serious emotional problem, necessitates deeper study even when the question of abuse does not arise, if another 'accident' is to be prevented. A comparatively small number of patients (12.5 per cent) in a carefully documented general practice (McGregor 1969) became involved in a large proportion of accidents (30 per cent). The younger children suffered from lack of parental care and often one or other parent had had multiple accidents. Those involved in multiple accidents had double the sickness rate of the rest of the community.

Is the risk of accident evenly distributed? A study of childhood accidents in the 6- to 11-year-old group led Langford and his colleagues (1953) to describe three types of patient: (1) the over-active, restless, impulsive, whose control breaks down under stress; (2) the immature, lacking parental supervision and insisting on a degree of independence which they cannot support; and (3) hostile, resentful children. No general agreement yet exists that 'delinquency and accidents are both forms (or consequences) of deviant behaviour' (Meyer and Klein 1968), yet the magnitude of the accident problem in death, injury, hospitalization and loss of education merits its intensive study.

Injuries can be classified according to outcome as fatal or non-fatal, or with complete functional recovery or life-long handicap. A second type of classification relates to the kind of accident; the external cause: burns, scalds, poisoning, suffocation, drowning, falls, road vehicular, either as passenger or pedestrian. A third method describes the pathological lesion in the child, the nature of the injury: whether loss of tissue, shock, fracture, bruise, haemorrhage, brain damage, emotional disturbance. All of these classifications have as their starting point the moment of the accident. To be concerned with the accident and with what follows is practical and important, but insufficient. Prevention must, of course, take account of the nature of the accident and of 'safety' measures and devices and for this, epidemiological research and studies of the social environment have brought enlightenment. Yet, despite what is done, accidents still rank high in the causes of disablement and death. Enough psychological and behavioural observations have already been made to show that for prevention to be really effective, large-scale research is needed into all the processes that precede and predispose to the accident. This must include the emotional antecedents. And scientific meaning must be given to the diagnosis of 'accident prone'.

The accident service should have close links with both the paediatric department and the department of hygiene and preventive medicine, and should join in discussion and research with the department of psychological medicine. Because of the important part played by accident in mortality and morbidity, the subject should be given a bigger place in undergraduate training. Aetiology must first be thoroughly explored. Secondly, the lessons learned from these studies must be translated from polite recommendations in reports to action. Great expense is incurred in institutions because fire precautions officers demand fire escapes. But providing a fire escape does not make an institution or a family home safe. The money is totally wasted unless there is a fire and the money might be more effectively spent on non-inflammable building materials and clothes as well as safe heating appliances. Poisonous substances, whether prescribed drugs, cosmetics or cleaning materials, should be inaccessible to adventurous toddlers. Stairs and playspace should be as safe as they can be made. Parents should know about the emotional antecedents of accident.

Accidents that escape prevention need a varied programme of care. Among the 833 773 accidents involving school children in 1968, a figure compatible with the Newcastle prediction, 82 per cent were treated either by the general practitioner or as hospital out-patients (682 594). The school treated 7 per cent (58 364) while 2 per cent required no 'treatment' (19 675). Hospital in-patient treatment was needed by 9 per cent (75 031). HIPE for 1971 records discharges and deaths on account of fractures, wounds, contusions, concussion, foreign bodies, burns and nerve injuries under 5 years of age as 43 937, and 70 800 from 5 to 14 years. This is a formidable total of 114 737 children. The total childhood deaths from all kinds of accidents in 1971 amounted to 2122.

The pathological lesions caused by accidents call for the services of many special units within any accident service. The most common apart from the general treatment for shock and haemorrhage are those of the orthopaedic unit, while for the most serious the need is the burns unit and the plastic surgery and the neurosurgical services. The emotional stresses of a serious accident and its complex prolonged and unpleasant treatment are especially important for children. The effect on one or both parents may be intense because they may have been responsible by act of omission or commission and they may feel the heavy guilt of this responsibility. They may also be rightly anxious about the immediate and long-term results. A place should be found for the psychiatrist and the social worker. In a long drawn out course of treatment and rehabilitation, the educationist should not be left out.

Available figures allow the total accidents to be broken down into five main sub-divisions, road traffic accidents, and accidents in the home, which are further divided into suffocation, falls, poisonings, and burns and scalds. In 1971 deaths due to water transport accidents numbered 20, to accidental drowning and submersion 230, to accident caused by electric current 26, and to self-inflicted injury and suicide 4. Homicide caused 97 deaths, 68 under the age of 5 years, 38 before the first birthday. The means are unspecified in 55. Sudden death, cause unknown, is included (ICD 795) under Class XVI, 'symptoms and ill-defined conditions'. It is as difficult to doubt that some of the 250 recorded deaths in RGSR 1971 were accidental as that some were due to deliberate act.

COT DEATHS, SUDDEN UNEXPECTED DEATH IN INFANTS (SUD)

Sudden infant deaths syndrome (SIDS)

Valdes-Dapena (1967) reviewed the world literature from 1954 to 1966 on this difficult but important subject, concluding that the medical profession remains 'woefully ignorant'. Incidence has been variously estimated between 1.4 (Ministry of Health 1965) and 3 per 1000 live births (Froggatt *et al.* 1971). Applying these figures to 1971 would give between 1096 and 2349 deaths of infants, three-quarters between one and six months of age. However, the total number of accidental deaths of all kinds was only 2122 with 261 deaths during these months. Another 220 deaths in the first six months are recorded as sudden death, cause unknown (ICD 795) including sudden unexpected death in infancy. Naturally the point of view of the observer makes a great difference and especially how satisfied he is to exclude cases where any other possibility can be found. Richards and McIntosh (1972) in Glasgow accepted 47 out of the 226 consecutive infant deaths studied but excluded 16 with the diagnosis of aspiration of gastric contents which many regard as agonal, a result of dying, and only exceptionally as a cause of death.

14 of these 16 and all the sudden unexpected deaths happened at home. Gardner and his colleagues (1967) have observed that respiratory syncytial virus and epiglottitis due to hemophilus infections may easily escape recognition. Accurate incidence estimates are only likely to be made when some clear definition has been agreed and then only when a special survey is conducted of all the infant deaths in a specified population area by a team of pathologists, virologists and epidemiologists with special experience. This is surely a child health need of some urgency, which is being investigated under the auspices of the Foundation for the Study of Infant Deaths.

From the viewpoint of prevention, evidence exists about contributory factors. The condition is commonest in the winter months, in twins, in disadvantaged families living in crowded dwellings, in young mothers with higher parities. No evidence points to an epidemic or a genetic incidence, but the siblings of propositi are at five times the risk of the general population (Froggatt *et al.* 1971).

Vaughan (1968) in a Salford general practice found a similar background. He noted in his 16 families that 12 had serious domestic problems and that in all but one some departure from the normal had been noted in the baby within days of death. The doctor had been called to 7 families. Emotional deprivation has been blamed, but so have such definite physical processes as allergy to cow's milk and a 'diving reflex' leading to ventricular fibrillation.

Once more, better environmental conditions and better 'mothering' would be expected to reduce the incidence of this important cause of infant death. Clinicians will all be aware of sudden unexplained infant deaths in the highest social and economic classes. They will also have had experience of incomplete resuscitation which has prolonged a life without restoring intelligence.

POISONING

The accidents due to poisoning seem, on the surface, to be the most easily preventable. They accounted for 29 266 hospital discharges and deaths in 1971, and to 158 deaths. Poisoning had been by medicinal substances in 65.9 per cent, a group contributing 17 per cent of the deaths. The relatively few deaths suggest that either hospital treatment is highly effective or that the poisoning was not of a very serious nature. The exception to either explanation is carbon monoxide poisoning with 120 deaths and 22 discharges and deaths in HIPE. Only 7 of these deaths were listed as due to accidental poisoning by carbon monoxide, when deaths were classified according to external cause rather than to nature of injury. The majority were due to accidents from 'fire and flames'.

Correlating HIPE with the deaths in RGSR gives an incomplete picture because a child dying from carbon monoxide poisoning at home would not ordinarily be admitted to hospital. In a survey of poisoning in children during the years 1965–69 inclusive, 'fires and explosions' were identified as causing two thirds of the deaths from carbon monoxide and only 16 per cent of these died in hospital. A case could be made for excluding carbon monoxide from the list of poisons on the grounds of a fundamental difference in the character of the accident. Motor vehicle accidents were responsible for 2 carbon monoxide deaths, and suicide and non-accidental poisoning for 36. Deaths relating to heating and cooking accidents occurred in 52 and to fires and explosions in 125 in the 5-year period.

Non-medicinal substances accounted for almost one half of the total poisoning, and among the groups, each of which causes the annual discharge from hospital of more than 1000, are corrosives, acids and alkalis (1628) with a high proportion of bleaching solutions, industrial solvents (1595) especially turpentine, and petroleum products (1384) largely paraffin. Deaths from these accidents are infrequent, but there are long-term effects of caustic soda on the oesophagus and of paraffin on the lungs, which require considerable and prolonged hospital treatment and which cannot be identified from the statistical tables. For example hospital discharges and deaths from diseases of the oesophagus amount to 399, with 19 deaths mainly within the first year and therefore unlikely to be due to a draught of caustic fluid. The toxic effects of lead and its compounds in 1971 are blamed for only 44 discharges and deaths and 2 RGSR deaths. This is much less than the 200 diagnosed cases each year suggested by Hospital Activity Analysis (Barltrop 1971) and very much less than the 2000 per annum arrived at by extrapolation from a small area (56 homes) on the basis of hazard through exposure to old lead paint (Barltrop and Killala 1969). Much depends on whether exposure to lead and a relatively small rise in the blood lead level is taken seriously in a child without specific symptoms. Lead encephalopathy with its serious and irreversible character is fortunately rare, but Hernberg and Nikkanen (1970) have shown inhibition by lead of some enzyme activity and Millar *et al.* (1970) have drawn attention to decreased enzyme activity in the brain (amino-laevulinic acid dehydratase, ALA) so that environmental pollution by lead causing sub-clinical disease in young children should perhaps be taken more seriously. Positive efforts should be made to remove lead paint from old houses, which is the usual source of lead.

Noxious food stuffs (1805) and 'other non-medicinal substances' (2801) also account for many presumed preventable hospital admissions and no doubt represent only a fraction of a total which includes many treated at home by the family doctor or even by the mother on her own.

Cosmetic toxicity seldom produces serious results although the ingestion of face creams, lipsticks, skin lotions and other dressing table chemicals produces considerable maternal anxiety. The composition of these materials and their potential danger to children need to be kept under review and ought in future to be included in any scheme concerned with the safety of drugs.

The largest numbers of admissions for poisoning by medicinal substances results from salicylate. In the 1965–69 study this was estimated as 5000 annual admissions, 90 per cent in the 1- to 4-year age group and 73 per cent being due to aspirin. HIPE estimates 7973 discharges and deaths from analgesics and antipyretics (RGSR deaths 8). Other substances accounting for over 1000 are psychotherapeutic agents (2325), 'other' sedatives (1129), agents primarily affecting the autonomic nervous system (941) and 'other unspecified drugs' (3565).

Health needs

Enumeration of the deaths suggests that the treatment of suspected or established poisoning is well carried out through the casualty departments assisted by the five capital city government sponsored Poisons Information Centres and the three others in Leeds, Manchester and Newcastle. The Hill Report (1968) recommended a poisoning treatment centre in each district general hospital with at least one consultant with a special interest. Appropriate laboratory facilities should be available. In practice the centre would be best sited in the Accident and Emergency Centre which, ideally, would have staff and treatment arrangements suitable for children and infants, a close link with the hospital children's department and with the psychiatric department. The Hill Report draws attention to the need for the ambulance service to have precise instructions about what to do and personnel and facilities to do it.

The Hill Report also states that 'We think that the majority of deaths from poisoning in children are avoidable'. Is the poisoning itself avoidable? They note the similarity of some drugs or pills to sweets and the needs of the toddler to explore the environment. Matthew (1972) stresses the duty of parents to store drugs in cupboards inaccessible to children and locked, and urges doctors to press for safety packaging of drugs.

The extra cost would be offset many times by the saving of hospital beds.

In introducing the subject, Matthew classified poisoning as suicidal, accidental, manipulative and homicide, which last he notes as very rare. With the exception of the truly accidental, motives in the rest can be very strong and strong enough to overcome considerable difficulties of access. Children do not often attempt suicide, but they are very interested in manipulative activities which play on the emotions of their parents. There is also a strong possibility that poison may be one of the weapons used by parents in child abuse*. To be effective, methods of prevention must be informed by a deep knowledge of true causation. Locking the medicine cupboard and keeping household cleaning fluids and other dangerous substances out of the reach of young children must help, but much study is needed, especially on the emotional and psychological sides, before there is the full understanding which gives the only hope of effective prevention.

Doctors as well as parents can be responsible for introducing toxic substances to their child patients. Retrolental fibroplasia and blindness from oxygen therapy and kernicterus from the hyperbilirubinaemia induced by large doses of vitamin K are but two dramatic examples. The prescriber must be ever on guard against the harmful effects on drug metabolism of delayed maturation of enzyme systems in the newborn and of genetic abnormalities in some older individuals.

It should be noted that adult self-poisoning, the *cri de coeur*, has a definite relationship to childhood in a broken home (Kessel 1965).

ROAD TRAFFIC ACCIDENTS

The HIPE analysis of road traffic accidents totalling 19 050 with 4500 under 5 years and 14 550 between 5 and 15 years gives 240 discharges and deaths and RGSR records 26 deaths in the first year of life. The largest single group is for intra-cranial injury (without skull fracture), 7380 in the 5- to 14-year group forming about half of the total in this group and 38.7 per cent of all road traffic accident discharges and deaths during childhood. By the age of 3 years there is a marked preponderance of boys over girls. These accidents caused 586 deaths in children of 5 to 14 years, 22.6 per cent of the 2593 total deaths in the age group. By contrast deaths from accidents in the home and residential institutions were commonest in the 0- to 4-year age group providing 557 out of a total of 660 among children under 15 years old. Whose is the responsibility for protecting the child from the dangers in the home and

* See Rogers, D., Tripp, J., Bentovim, A. et al., Brit. Med. J., 1976, 1, 793–6

in the streets? Presumably reliance must be placed on parents in the first instance and an important part of parenting must always be the protection of children from common dangers. The responsibility ought to be better discharged if parents were really made aware of what the dangers are and how they may be avoided. At school the teachers have the opportunity to teach children about accidents. Whatever is done, and probably much more positive teaching effort could be made, two other problems remain.

The first is how far the community takes the responsibility for insisting on increased public safety. Heating, lighting and other power operated household apparatus can be safe or dangerous. The sale of inflammable building and other materials including plastic and clothing could be regulated. So could containers for dangerous drugs and non-medicinal chemical substances. The provision of adequate playspace, adequate both in quantity and quality, could be one of the community's responsibilities. It is a curious reflection on our sense of values and priorities that so much law and effort goes into the control of property and material possessions, while great areas of danger to child life and health remain uncontrolled. The dangers are known. So too are technical preventive measures. The matter seems to be of insufficient importance to weigh the balance in favour of child health needs when on the other side are costs and changes of method and habit.

The second problem concerns the character of the child. From the earliest hours of its life the baby is driven to take risks. That they are not knowingly taken does not reduce the risk element of new achievement. This becomes obvious when the infant begins exploring the world of its home, but risk has been inherent in earlier attempts at movement. It becomes even more obvious when the child starts to drive a motor car, and at this stage society intervenes with the command to take a course of instruction, obtain a licence and remain thereafter under more or less police surveillance. That this is not the whole answer is shown by the toll of road traffic accidents and deaths. But, although present methods are not wholly successful, it would be a bold man who would deny that the situation would be much graver without them or that defects of character and of emotional control play a large part in the causation of road traffic accidents. Better planning and lighting of roads, although costly, could also play a part. A clinical approach to the aetiology of childhood accidents with its regard for careful history taking and its enquiry into the details of family life would be revealing and might form the basis for a more rational and perhaps a more effective accident prevention service.

Health needs

No less than 11 per cent of all children in maintained schools in England and Wales have at least one accident in a year according to the Report on the Health of the School Child, 1966–68, which points out that accidents are now responsible for one third of all deaths in this school population. The Newcastle observers predict a significant accident for one out of every ten children each year, a grand total of over 800 000 (0 to 14 years). In the NCB cohort 20 per cent had been admitted to hospital because of some kind of accident between birth and the seventh birthday.

Deaths from accidents of all kinds (RGSR 1971) before the fifteenth birthday numbered 2122 with the expected preponderance of males at all ages (1384 M to 738 F). As many as 21 per cent had occurred before the first birthday, 29.5 per cent before the second and 51.7 per cent before the age of 5 years. The major risks in the first year of life are suffocation or obstruction from inhalation or ingestion of food or other objects or from mechanical suffocation which accounted for 297, 65.8 per cent of the total 451. The bulk of road traffic deaths come between the second and the tenth birthdays (524 out of a total of 819). Much fewer in numbers are deaths from accidents caused by fire and flames (138) and by falls (135). As would be expected these affect mostly the children under 5 and especially those under 2 years old.

These mortality figures are serious enough. They do not reveal the numbers of children permanently disabled. In the NCB cohort 16 children had died as the result of accident by the age of 7 years, and 31 were left with a serious disability. That is to say that of those admitted to hospital for treatment of accident 0.5 per cent had died and 1.0 per cent were left seriously disabled ($n = 3000$).

The health needs of children in relation to accidents concern the whole family, prevention being of prime importance. The general public has learned to expect childhood accidents as inevitable experiences with the same resignation with which they once accepted diphtheria, measles and anterior poliomyelitis. More is known today about measures that could be taken to prevent accidents to children than was known 50 years ago about the prevention of these infections. Yet these are no longer risks. If the community really willed, the environment could now be made safer for children by giving its proper high priority to accident prevention.

NON-ACCIDENTAL TRAUMA AND CHILD ABUSE

Although deliberate trauma cannot properly be regarded as accidental, nevertheless this important and disturbing subject must be included in the section on accidents. The first reason is that the injured baby or child is likely to present to the family doctor with a history of accident, albeit not always an entirely convincing one, or to the Accident and Emergency Department of the hospital. The second is that, as has already been suggested, many of the forms of injury labelled accidental, while not deliberate, are probably not entirely fortuitous. Accidental and non-accidental trauma become more closely allied as knowledge grows about both.

Prevalence: Until reporting becomes a statutory obligation, prevalence cannot be known and statutory reporting requires some form of definition. In the United States the concept of child abuse includes as well as physical injury, neglect, malnutrition other than by accidental means and the deliberate withholding of food. The width of this concept, which would seem both necessary and wise, explains the high rate now suggested. Kempe (personal communication 1974) expects a prevalence rate of 380 per million total population. Some variation exists between the different states of the Union but little between urban and rural communities in a given state. With a population in England and Wales of approximately 48.5 million (1971), reporting should reveal between 18 000 and 19 000 children each year. Kempe's earlier estimated incidence (1971) of 6 per 1000 live births would have produced 4700 in 1971, a figure that more nearly approximates to Malcolm Hall's projection (1975) of 4400 from his fairly complete studies in Preston. Given a wide definition and experience of reporting, prevalence estimates would be bound to increase and as the main cause for such an increase would be the inclusion of the less severely injured and more of the neglected children, mortality rates would tend to decrease. Kempe gives 5 per cent as the current US figure, which if applied with his prevalence figures to England and Wales would suggest the deaths of 920 children from child abuse every year. If the Preston mortality rate of 17.2 per cent were applied to Hall's suggested 4400 annual cases, there would be 750 deaths and even the more usually accepted mortality rate of 10 per cent gives as many as 450 deaths. If these deaths really do occur, and there is no good reason to doubt it, they are not identifiable in any statistics, official or unofficial. Only 97 deaths in children are recorded in RGSR (1971) as due to homicide or purposeful injury with a further 49 classified as 'not certain if inflicted'. There are in addition 250 'sudden deaths cause unknown' under the age of 4 years. But death is not always the sequel.

A number of observers have drawn attention to serious neurological sequelae with an incidence as high as one third and with sub-dural haematoma, cerebral palsy, mental handicap and visual impairment as the most serious. The nature of the permanent damage does depend upon the age of the child. The severe shaking of a baby in the first six months of life is the probable cause of sub-dural haematoma and of vascular damage within the brain itself as well as of retinal haemorrhage and blindness. Follow-up examinations of shaken babies showed a surprisingly high incidence of mental handicap. Mac Keith (1975) has suggested that these injuries may be responsible for as many as 400 new brain injured children each year, 'a sizeable proportion of the unexplained cases of cerebral palsy and mental deficiency'.

Besides these gross physical sequels, the effects of deprivation on growth of body and mind and on the personality and the learning ability of the sufferer must be taken into account. Long-term observation is essential if the facts are ever to be known.

Health needs

This problem causes increasing concern among paediatricians and all family social workers. The aims are clear, to prevent child abuse in the first place and, if this does not succeed, to protect the children in the families involved from both repeated injury and chronic deprivation. The general practitioner may expect to encounter one family in five years and therefore to have little chance of becoming experienced in diagnosis. His suspicions should be aroused when a family keeps seeking attention for trivial episodes, especially when they include bruises, lacerations, cigarette burns or unaccountable failure to thrive. Despite obvious anxiety, the parents may delay a call or a visit for a surprising length of time after an 'incident' and the story may not only be inconsistent with the actual lesions found, but vary when retold. It would be wise for the attached health visitor to make an investigation into the family's environment and inter-personal relationships under these circumstances, but wiser still if she was so engaged for all 'accidents' to young children in the practice.

When there is real suspicion of abuse or of deliberate trauma, the urgent need is for admission to a paediatric department or hospital for full assessment and diagnosis. A careful history, a blood examination to exclude a disorder of coagulation, a skeletal survey and photographs are essential. This investigation can only be made in hospital. At the same time a family investigation is required, both socio-economic and psychological. It cannot be stressed too strongly that the management of the family demands team work. Hospital and community social workers contribute to the full assessment on which diagnosis rests, and social service departments have the statutory duty to protect children in their area. Child abuse is a crime and the police have a legal obligation to investigate crime. The help of the Juvenile Court Magistrates is often needed for a place of safety or care order, so that parents' panic withdrawal of their baby from the safety of the hospital can be controlled.

Paediatricians have a duty to see themselves, not as directors of management, but as members of a true team; they must do their best to ensure in the area in which they work that case conferences are called on suspicion and that its members are imbued with a team spirit. The hospital doctor, the social services and the police, together with the general practitioner and the practice health visitor are basic members. The paediatrician's responsibility is also to deal with the Courts himself, or to encourage a local doctor with legal experience, such as a police surgeon, or an appointed senior member of his staff to handle this side of the work. An inexperienced junior member unable to stand up to defence counsel or a clever solicitor may fail to impress the Court with the result that the baby returns home to be killed or maimed in due time. The Magistrate's Court can only reach a decision on the evidence presented to it.

The paediatrician should also establish working policies with the accident and emergency or the casualty departments, so that a senior doctor is always called in for discussion when even the remotest possibility of deliberate trauma exists. Arrangements must vary from hospital to hospital, but especial care is called for when casualty officers are inexperienced, serve for short periods only or have language difficulties.

Much education is still needed to alert all who may be concerned that, in non-accidental injury, minor lesions, for example, facial bruising or small burns produced by lighted cigarettes, are in reality major warnings of the risk to life that the baby runs. To what extent education in family health in schools would prevent the trouble is unknown. In between 10 and 30 per cent of the families, the father is an aggressive psychopath, and many mothers are of below average intelligence. Psychopathic or severely psychotic parents cannot be trusted not to injure their children. At least in these families discussions with Family Planning clinics are important. Many of the parents are known to have had a deprived childhood or to have been injured by their own parents. This fact stresses the need for preventive means. Prison sentences may not help rehabilitation.

The best interest of the children will be served if certain principles guide conduct:

1 complete co-operation is essential with mutual respect between all professional workers involved;
2 one individual should not make the decision which needs a 'team' of at least two from two different disciplines;
3 full assessment and full information are necessary prerequisites to any management decisions;
4 the therapeutic team must never be the team which assesses the success or failure of the management. One individual must relate to and take responsibility for handling the family but must always refer back to the decision-making team;
5 as far as possible the original case conference should recognize the group of 'incurable' parents so that long-term plans for alternative care for the children are not delayed. Aggressive psychopaths, some schizophrenics and some parents with unrealistic ideas of child behaviour are not to be trusted with the care of children;
6 help for family rehabilitation has to be viewed widely and includes detailed attention to the living problems of the family. Deprivation can also be iatrogenic.

If the paediatrician and his staff are to apply these principles in practice, much time will be consumed, and this must be remembered when staff requirements are being considered. Kempe estimates that one team is needed for every 300 000 to 400 000 population and that is 150 teams for England and Wales. The whole time of one paediatrician, preferably made up from the part time services of more than one, would be required. Some work will undoubtedly fall to the paediatrician's lot, at least in teaching, in relation to the provision of 'aids', mothers' groups, crisis nurseries, therapeutic day school, if not for periodic personal discussions with the families. The rehabilitation of families will not be as successful as it should be without these provisions. The whole enterprise of care for these sick families is coming to occupy more and more of the time of paediatricians. As the abused child may present to resident hospital staff of all kinds as well as to general practitioners, the subject should certainly be included in the general undergraduate syllabus.

CHAPTER 20

Stressful situations

Stress is not always bad for a family or for the children within the family. A challenge accepted and met with fortitude and faith can bring out qualities in a family that would otherwise have lain dormant. At a time when services are limited, pairs of helping hands scarce and money in short supply, the spotlight of attention must be turned on to the vulnerable and assistance to go to those who are so vulnerable that the risk is real that stress will lead to family or personal breakdown. Certain family situations are generally accepted as stressful. It would seem wise therefore to ensure that special regard be paid to the children in these dangerous situations.

Unfortunately two trends in current social philosophy oppose such selectivity. First of all is the view that fairness interpreted as equality over-rides all else. Therefore either everyone has what is offered or no-one should have it. The second trend is to encourage fantasy at the expense of truth. The sections in this chapter concern children in care, adoption, one parent families and drug dependent children. Everyone knows that children in care suffer deprivation by comparison with children happily ensconced within their own families. Yet society as a whole acts in the belief that it has done its best and discharged its duty, the problem solved, when a child is taken into care and that society need not examine too closely what follows.

With regard to adoption, the fantasy begins with the conception and little insight is needed to observe distortion at every stage, the mother's view of her pregnancy, the hopes of the adopters for both themselves and the child, and later the child's own search for identity. As to families that are one-parent by choice, the ultimate fantasy is that to have a husband is unnatural and that the word 'daddy' must be expunged from the language, including Janet and John reading books. Views on the wisdom of making 'soft' drugs available are mixed and many are able to find satisfactory arguments for adding to socially accepted alcohol and tobacco this further stumbling block to health.

The preceding paragraphs may seem to some exaggerated or even irrelevant. In defence it must be claimed that the truth, the realities of situations are of importance because the proffered solutions cannot succeed unless they are directed at those realities. Accurate diagnosis is an essential prelude to proper treatment. The beliefs of doctors, health visitors, social workers as well as of legislators and administrators, are both powerful and relevant in the discharge of their various functions.

CHILDREN IN CARE

The number of children under the age of 18 years in England and Wales 'in care' on 31 March 1971 was 87 377 representing 6.5 per 1000 of the population 0 to 18 years. During the earlier peak years in 1966 and 1967 the numbers were little short of 80 000 and the prevalence 6.1 and 6.0 per 1000. The number coming into care during 1971 was 64 545.

The effect of the open breakdown of family life is not the same for the baby, the infant and the child. Neverthless a stable family life is generally assumed to be one of the main requirements for the growth, development and health of all children. The single fact of being in care does not create a homogeneous group, and therefore a study of morbidity, mortality and disorders of behaviour among children in care cannot be expected to produce figures comparable with those from the whole child population.

Except for sudden, accidental death of one or both parents, the 'into care' decision is the culmination of a process which has been placing a strain upon all the members of the family for a longer or a shorter time. The child is not suddenly losing a complete and happy life. The current tables published by the Home Office list the reasons why the child came into care, the age grouping and the reason why children went out of care during the year. The number of deaths with an analysis of 'cause' and age used to be recorded, and would have been of greater value if the 'cause' had been related to age and to the duration of care. The largest single reason for taking into care is short-term illness of parent or guardian (16 004) and the third is confinement of the mother (5235) (see Table 20.1). These two groups total 21 257 and, although stressful events for the children, should not have led to long-term harmful effects of themselves, that is to say unless the child was already in an unstable condition.

The second largest group follows desertion by the mother (5487) with a few (699) where the mother has died and the father cannot cope. There follows illegitimacy when mother cannot provide a home (2436). Home and housing conditions were responsible for 6126 (unsatisfactory home conditions 3176, homeless through eviction 1441 and through other reasons 1555). Conflict with the law by parents or by child account for almost 7000, raising all the questions about relationships between psychological and mental health and housing and socio-economic conditions.

Table 20.1. Number of children who came into care in England and Wales 1st April 1970 to 31st March 1971 (HMSO Cmmd. 5100)

Because of :			
Short-term illness of parent or guardian	16 004		21 257
Confinement of mother	5 235		
Desertion of mother	5 487		
Illegitimacy	2 436		
Unsatisfactory home conditions	3 176		6 162
Homeless (evicted 1 441)	2 996		
Long-term illness of parent or guardian	1 293		
Absence or desertion, of both parents, death of mother	1 695		
Imprisonment or remand in custody of parent or guardian	1 028		
Fit person orders : offenders	12 328		
non-offenders	6 998		
Matrimonial Causes Act	465		
All other reasons	5 395		
Grouped by age:	on coming into care 1970–1	in care	
under two years	11 049	4 377	
two to five years	12 376	8 951	
of compulsory school age	29 474	49 968	
over compulsory school age	11 646	24 081	
Total	64 545	87 377	

Almost one third (30.6 per cent) came into care during the sensitive pre-school years (under 5 years) when the foundations are being laid for successful education.

The list of reasons why the children went out of care shows that the majority (39 043) were transferred to 'parent, guardian, relative or friend', while some (4430) became independent at 18 years, and a small and declining group were adopted (1870). The pattern of the 1116 notified deaths in 1969 presented no remarkable features.

Of all the 87 377 children in care of local authorities in England and Wales on 31 March 1971, 41.3 per cent were boarded out and another 51.3 per cent were in some form of residential home, nursery or school. In the absence of precise and contrary evidence all these children must be assumed to be under the stress of family breakdown, whether temporary or permanent.

For half of them it is likely to be permanent and this stress is added to a period of varying length during which family life has been through problems of emotion, accident or disease heading for collapse. The children should therefore receive every help which the community can provide in the way of preventive medical services, and their health should be recognized as a personal responsibility by an appropriate team of doctors and social workers. A link with the children in long-stay hospital accommodation might be practicable in some areas through the area review committees brought into existence to help with the problems of child abuse. This is of special importance for those children for whom no chance remains of a return to the security of normal family life.

A serious deprivation, included in the Home Office list, results from the death of the mother when the father cannot cope, of whom 699 were taken into care. The total number of live babies left motherless through obstetric death cannot be discovered from the periodic reports 'On Confidential Enquiries into Maternal Deaths in England and Wales'. The latest report (HMSO 1972) records for 1967–69 698 maternal deaths (28.4 per 100 000 maternities).

Table 20.2. Maternal deaths in 2 457 440 Maternities England and Wales 1967–9
Pregnancy and childbirth

	Direct cause	*Associated cause*
Deaths	455	248
Rate per 100 000	18.5	9.9

It is interesting that in a report aimed at prevention, the concentration is so intense on the circumstances of the reasons for death in pregnancy, that there is no compartment for the baby.

ADOPTION

Adoption is a legal process which sometimes involves doctors. In connexion with health needs the fact that a child is adopted indicates one thing only, that he should be given a careful medical examination in order that adopting parents may be aware of any problem that might affect their method of management and the child's future. Three other facts are important. These are whether one or other parent is the adopter, whether the birth was 'out of wedlock' with the resulting social problem, and the child's age at the time of adoption.

Most of the medical safeguards which complicate adoption plans centre round the adoption of illegitimate babies by parents unrelated to them and soon after birth before their physical, intellectual and emotional potential can be confidently predicted. By contrast, the greatest difficulties in placing arise over the adoption of older children with severe handicaps who may well be legitimate, but who have suddenly lost their parents. Belonging to a minority race or religion increases the difficulty.

Table 20.3. Illegitimate live births

	Males	Totals Females	Persons	Deaths under 1 year	Under 1 yr. death rate per 1000 live births Illeg.	Leg.
1963	30 220	28 884	59 104	1 536	26.00	21.13
1964	32 727	30 613	63 340	1 665	26.00	19.92
1965	34 080	32 169	66 249	1 649	24.89	19.00
1966	34 386	32 670	67 056	1 646	24.55	19.00
1967	35 784	34 144	69 928	1 655	23.67	19.00
1968	35 815	33 991	69 806	1 632	23.38	18.29
1969	34 401	32 640	67 041	1 721	25.65	18.04
1970	33 279	31 465	64 744	1 693	26.15	18.19
1971	33 961	31 717	65 678	1 669	25.41	17.52
1972	32 313	30 198	62 511	1 408	22.52	17.23

During 1971, adoption orders were made for 21 495 children, 14 907 illegitimate and 6588 legitimate, with a slight preponderance of boys. The majority of the legitimate children were adopted into their own families, almost all after the age of 2 years, so that their medical care should have differed in no way from that of the general child population. But even among the illegitimate children only a little over half were adopted in the first year (52 per cent) and more than 1 in 8 after the age of 2 years. At the most, then, about 8000 babies during the year needed special examination and assessment from the point of view of adoption. On the other hand illegitimate children who are not adopted and who either remain in the care of unsupported unmarried mothers or who are brought up in foster homes or institutions run all the risks to normal development of children deprived of a complete family life. The possibility that the health needs of these children have been underestimated is discussed later. Some of these children are likely to be among those adopted late in childhood.

The numerical relationship between adoptions and illegitimacy is not absolute. Between 1957 and the peak year 1968 the actual numbers of illegitimate births doubled and the number of adoption orders also reached a peak of 24 831. Birth rate, which began its decline in 1964, illegitimacy rate and the number of adoption orders have all dropped since. The reasons, like the reasons for their earlier rise, rest in the realms of theory, so that prediction would be unwise. In 1971 the illegitimacy rate was 83.8 per 1000 live births, 65 678 out of 783 155. Making the artificial assumption that all babies adopted in their first 12 months can be regarded as 1971 babies, adoption was arranged for only 22.7 per cent of the illegitimate babies.

The initial examination of the baby for whom adoption is being arranged is not to determine suitability for adoption as has sometimes wrongly been supposed, but to identify any defects, so that adopters may have the fullest possible information about the physical condition of the baby. This examination should be carried out by a paediatrician or physician with neonatal experience or by a general practitioner or physician from the local authority service who has made himself thoroughly familiar with assessment in the first year of life. Unfortunately, the statement is still made by some doctors that they will be 'unable to sign the baby up' for a period of months, as if they were expected to certify the baby as 'normal' or 'abnormal', whereas their duty is to do no more than state the history and the observations upon the baby that result from the examination. It is for the medical adviser and for the adoption agency itself to discuss placement with a would-be adopter in the light of all this information.

The question of the inheritance from the mother and the putative father of diseases, particularly of mental disorder, or of propensities towards anti-social or criminal behaviour, is often raised. Many gaps exist in exact knowledge of these risks, about which there are strongly held prejudices, and genetic counselling should be available and employed by adoption agencies when these questions arise.

Babies for adoption are referred to in the section on screening for metabolic and other inherited diseases as a special group for whom these methods may be advisable. At present a blood test for syphilis is common and a test for phenylketonuria is the rule. The reasons for this extra caution are not far to seek. With few exceptions the couples who are prepared to welcome the adoption of an unrelated baby do so because they are unable to produce offspring of their own. This is itself a source of strain. The unexpected discovery that the adopted baby is mentally handicapped or suffering from a serious disability such as cerebral palsy or disease which needs prolonged and exacting treatment like phenylketonuria, cystic fibrosis, haemophilia or muscular dystrophy may prove too great a burden.

Couples judged suitable to act as adopters of other people's children should be able to deal with problems like haemangiomas, benign cardiac murmurs or peculiarities in the shape of the feet. For babies and children with serious abnormalities there is a special need for the chance to develop within a secure, accepting and loving family circle. Perhaps the population capable of providing for these needs differs from the population from which have come the traditional adopters who may be seeking compensation for something lacking in their own lives. Because of the importance to growing children of the security of family life preventive medicine requires that this aspect of the adoption problem should be investigated. Recent studies have suggested that the adoption of older children has a greater success rate than has been generally supposed.

ONE-PARENT FAMILIES

Since the studies of Wynn published in 1964, the problems presented by fatherless families have been brought to the attention of the public. By identifying themselves as a group, at present a minority group, the lone parents have been able to exert political pressure, to obtain for themselves a special status in matters of social welfare and to have their plight made the subject of a committee under the chairmanship of the late Sir Morris Finer and at a cost of over £200 000.

The two-volume report of the Finer Committee contains a quantity of invaluable information and many recommendations that have a wider application than to the one-parent family. Legal, social welfare and educational illuminations abound. But with regard to any special child health needs, there is room for further study of the effects of upbringing in a one-parent family on general health, behaviour and school attainments.

The number of these incomplete families is steadily increasing, from 1968 to 1972 by 38 per cent (Finer 1974). The latest figure is of some quarter of a million. The mother's marital status in one-parent families receiving supplementary benefit in 1972 expressed as a percentage of the total 252 000 fatherless families, was separated 43.6, single 25, divorced 18.6, widowed 10.3 and prisoner's wife 2.4. There were an additional 7000 motherless families. The care of the children under the age of 5 years requires either that the parent is not in employment or raises the questions of baby minders and day nurseries, both of which have important medical implications.

It seems proper to regard the child of the one-parent family as a child with a degree of deprivation and therefore vulnerable to stress. His inclusion in this chapter is unlikely to be approved by members of the single parent pressure groups.

The widowed and prisoners' wives from only about 15 per cent of all one-parent families, while the separated where presumably both parents retain some responsibility for the children and where the greatest emotional tensions are expected provide 42 per cent. The biggest percentage increase from 1968 to 1972 has been of the divorced (64 per cent), with single next (42 per cent). By contrast the widowed have increased by only 6 per cent. Bearing in mind the amount of maladjustment and behaviour disturbance that produce symptoms for which doctors are consulted some of the conclusions of the Thousand Families Study (Miller *et al.* 1974) are worth restating. Disturbed behaviour and maladjustment were strongly related to unsatisfactory and variable relationships with the mother, while grandparents seldom appeared to play a causal role. There was a strong association between maladjustment and marital disharmony, and a clear association between severe maladjustment and gross family disturbance. Here surely is a problem of preventive health that needs to be explored.

This is a large and increasing group and if the numbers continue to increase by 38 per cent every four years, it would seem sensible to make some long-term observations so that child health needs can be recognized with a view to the provision of appropriate medical as well as social support.

Some legal implications

At some time in the remote future all legislation relating to the care of children and of their rights may be brought together in a consolidated act of parliament. If the health, mental and physical, of the nation's children were in fact regarded as part of the nation's capital, it would be at a time less remote. Meanwhile in relation to existing law, doctors, be they paediatricians, psychiatrists or general practitioners, are invited to give expert evidence to the courts. Much of what passes for expert opinion at present is not based on observations but rather on theory and the divergences of opinion revealed are duly exploited by the adversary system traditional in the law. The development of Family Courts in which an inquisitorial element complements the adversary system would lead in time to a change in the role of the expert from protagonist to assessor. The power of his unchallenged opinions would then increase. If doctors are to be used in this way, they must have at their command careful long-term studies of the effects of the sort of deprivation described in this chapter on the development of children.

Without this, the courts, in their dealings with breakdown of family life, will lack truly expert advice.

DRUG DEPENDENCE

The part played by the medical profession in the treatment of patients who have become drug dependent is undisputed and important. Few of the drug dependents are children under the age of 15 years. But has the child health profession any responsibility for contributing to prevention? Figures show that adolescence is an especially vulnerable period with its crisis of problems and of choices. Although the enthusiasms of adolescence share attributes with religious conversion and changes in behaviour may be dramatic and unexpected, it is difficult to believe that a normal, healthy, stable child will suddenly take to drugs in adolescence.

Unfortunately knowledge of the factors which favour and those which protect against drug dependence are lacking. As with accident prevention, the study which begins with the incident or with the recognition of the established drug dependence, is not sufficiently helpful. Reasons can be surmised, the novelty of a reputedly pleasurable experience, a holiday from educational or other pressures, an attempt to recapture a lost self-esteem, or a compulsion to identify with a group whose life-style includes drug taking. The only defences, while drugs remain available, are strength of character, experience in making 'good' choices and possibly a knowledge of the dangers and likely sequels, albeit danger can be one of the attractions.

Studies of youthful drug dependent populations have suggested that at least five intra-familial factors operate: the absence of a father, a domineering mother, hostility or conflict between parents, unreasonable parental aspirations for children and an absence in the family of the cultivation of any principles of behaviour or rules of life. Bransby *et al.* (1973) report that one third of the drug addicts born in England came from broken homes. The segregation of older children and adolescents in a learning state in school has created a new and artificial population that is a poor substitute for the apprenticeship during which the adolescent learned to work usefully in contact and in co-operation with respected adults. This new arrangement, which follows the lengthening of school days, may strengthen some innate adolescent reactions such as the rejection of traditions, the need to experiment, an unwillingness to accept a 'lecture for your own good' and, because of the discipline imposed by the school life, much of which appears unreasonable, both a lack of experience in making choices and antagonism to authority. Zacune and

Hensman (1971) conclude from their survey that 'at risk' groups include some 'who have already resisted attempts at formal education in other contexts'.

The doctor, general practitioner or paediatrician, who can view the development of children within the family, should be able to gather observations which will shed light on the factors which influence adolescent drug dependence even if he cannot yet alter attitudes. At least the paediatrician with community responsibility could begin by regarding the problem as one of his concerns. The subject is sufficiently important to be given a place in the paediatric curriculum. In 1967, 38 per cent of cannabis prosecutions (938 out of 2419) involved the age group 15 to 20 years (Wootton 1970). In 1968, 27 per cent of drug addicts known to the Home Office (Spear 1969) were under 20 years of age (764 out of 2782), and 9 out of 10 were heroin addicts (709). In a recent study of 666 drug addicts notified between March 1970 and December 1971 and taking heroin, methadone or cocaine, Bransby *et al.* (1973) found that 32 per cent were under 20 years old, one quarter had begun by the age of 17, and one third of those on amphetamines and cannabis had begun by the age of 15 years.

In a more direct way the doctor could examine critically the extent to which his own therapeutic responses have become drug dependent. He could, for example, measure the frequency with which he prescribes tranquillizers aimed at smothering the symptoms of malaise, of stress or of boredom, produced within families. Perhaps he begins with the baby who cries in the night. He might conclude that the medical profession shares with drug manufacturers some responsibility for encouraging men and women to solve their life problems through drugs and in so doing set an unwise example to the succeeding generation.

CHAPTER 21

Some problems of immigrant children

DEFINITION

Immigrant children are defined for statistical purposes as:

(i) all children born outside the British Isles now here with parents or guardians whose countries of origin were abroad, and
(ii) those born in the United Kingdom to parents whose countries of origin were abroad and who came here on or after 1 January, 10 years before the collection of information.

At 1 January 1970 the total number of immigrant children in the school population from under 5 to 19 years old exceeded a quarter of a million (263 710). Special tuition was required for 43 381 (16.4 per cent) and 4981 (1.9 per cent) were attending special schools. More than 40 per cent were West Indian and 29 per cent were Indian or Pakistanis. Table 21.1 shows the regions of their greatest distribution, their ethnic proportions and the trend towards increasing numbers, the 5–9-year-olds exceeding the 10–14-year-olds by 50 per cent.

Table 21.1. Immigrant school children (Jan. 1970)
(Statistics of education, vol. 1, Schools, HMSO 1971)

			per cent
Greater London	133 478	West Indian	41.7
West Midlands	42 118	Indian	19.8
Yorkshire and Humberside	17 731	Pakistani	9.2
East Midlands	15 597	12 others	39.3
6 other regions	54 786		
		5–9 years	138 811
Total	263 710	10–14 years	90 951
		Aged 5–14 years	229 762

Arthurton (1972) has discussed how in Bradford in 1969 the day-to-day work of the paediatrician was affected by the immigrant 7 per cent of the population. Asian (20 per cent) and negro (2 per cent) births accounted for 22 per cent of the total live births and for 12 per cent of the under-15-year-old population. Rhesus iso-immunization is rare. Language and cultural differences cause greater difficulties for the Asians than for negroes. The incidence of Asian low birth weight babies is almost double that of the indigenous population. History taking requires the presence of the father and examination of older female children by male doctors is unwelcome. Arthurton found in a random sample that only 20 per cent of Indian and 11 per cent of Pakistani mothers understood the doctor's instructions. The ratio of Asian in-patients (281) to total population was double that of others, the chief diagnoses being upper (57) and lower (38) respiratory infections and asthma (25). Poisoning and child abuse were no commoner among Asians, but attention is directed to tuberculosis, rickets and tropical diseases.

A speech therapist's report (Shields 1972) from Leeds comments on a high incidence of stammering among Pakistanis and Poles and of elective mutism in West Indians. Appointments are poorly kept and parents who lack skill in or are diffident about writing letters or using the telephone are unable to notify cancellations.

TUBERCULOSIS

The prevalence of childhood tuberculosis reflects the amount of infection in the adult population. This discussion, therefore, does not isolate children from adults. The heat treatment of liquid cow's milk is relied on to protect children from bovine infection. That there is a worldwide decline in notifications is established, but the level reached on the declining graph varies between one country and another. Immigration from a country of higher to one of lower prevalence is bound to affect notifications at least until the new citizens have adapted to the new environment. Differences in clinical presentation as well as in the site of infection have been noted. For example, Asians with pulmonary tuberculosis are less often sputum positive and the lesions are less extensive (McNichol *et al.* 1971). The proportion of non-respiratory tuberculosis, which is 10 per cent in the indigenous population, is 30 per cent in immigrants. The number of infected patients is twice as common among immigrants born in Eire and 4 to 6 times among Asian born immigrants as in the general population (Springett *et al.* 1958).

Table 21.2 gives the mean annual notifications in England and Wales, for three quinquennia, showing the decline.

Bignell (1971) has demonstrated an annual decline of some 9 per cent in tuberculosis notifications. His impeccable mathematics predict that in 1980 the rate in the school population will have dropped to 1 per

Table 21.2. Respiratory Tuberculosis
Mean annual notifications per 100 000 population England and Wales (from Springett 1972)

Years	*Aged* 0–4	5–14	15–29
1945	74	98	420
1955–59	55	53	218
1965–69	23	20	46

100 000. He foresees that with total annual notifications of no more than 1200, a special medical care service for tuberculosis will no longer be justified. In 1970 notifications were still 11 280 with 1465 deaths (Springett 1972). An influx of immigrants with active tuberculosis or with greater susceptibility than the indigenous population has altered the pattern without necessarily increasing the total number of notifications, so that optimism that there will be no long-term effect on the community seems justified. The risk, however, remains of family tragedies as the result of unexpected contact with open infection in school or at home.

In 1949–50 40.9 per cent of children aged 13 years were tuberculin positive. In 1970 the proportion had dropped to only 9 per cent. Springett in Birmingham has advocated chest radiography to identify infected immigrants and a greater use of BCG immunization to protect the school population. Doctors, health visitors and social workers in touch with Asian families could well encourage early BCG vaccination.

A general practitioner needs to be particularly alert when faced with an Asian-born immigrant with an illness lasting undiagnosed for more than a few days. Typhoid as Bignell points out, although occurring in only 2 per million of the population, holds an honoured place in differential diagnosis. Tuberculosis is apt to be forgotten. The mothers of young families should be critically regarded from this point of view.

If prevalence declines the general paediatrician of the future may well be expected to assume responsibility again for the management and care of the children infected with tuberculosis in the population which he serves.

Tuberculosis should remain one of the important subjects for general medical education. Particular reference should be made in instruction about the variation in prevalence, site and immunity responses of immigrant populations. In an area of high immigration, especially, but not exclusively by Asians, the questions of case finding and immunization should be discussed between the various members of the child health team.

RICKETS

Rickets has been the subject of several studies, in London, Birmingham and Rochdale since the peak period of immigration early in the last decade. Naturally workers in Glasgow, where infant rickets lingered longer among the indigenous population, were the first to herald its return (Arneil *et al*. 1963). And naturally the presence of skin pigmentation in this, as in so many problems of immigrants, has tended to cloud clear thinking. An early report of clinical rickets from south London (Benson *et al*. 1963) commented on skin pigmentation, but in fact only 7 of the 16 children were black. The prevalence of rickets with osteomalacia is greatest in areas of immigration from India and Pakistan, rather than from the West Indies. Swan and Cooke in Birmingham (1971) found two peaks, pubertal girls of average age 13.8 years and post-pregnancy women, the mothers of young families. Vaishnava and Rizvi (1971) point out that nutritional rickets is very common in India and is, in fact, the commonest metabolic bone disease seen in the large Irwin Hospital, New Delhi. A degree of under-nutrition and of anaemia judged by British standards is commonly associated. Among immigrants, the severity is not directly related to the length of stay in Britain, nor absolutely to the intake of calcium or phytic phosphorus. All improve when given calciferol.

The most recent study from Rochdale (Holmes *et al*. 1973) points to a possible constitutional difference between Asians and Caucasians in the metabolism of calciferol. Both cholecalciferol (D3) synthesized in the skin and ingested ergocalciferol (D2) are biologically inert precursors of the cholecalciferol elaborated in the liver. Synthesis and degradation depend on enzyme systems and these may differ in the two races. Neither severe nutritional disorder nor kwashiorkor has been diagnosed.

Children bring with them the *intestinal parasites* of their native land. They have no especial liability to become infested in Britain.

HEALTH NEEDS

Among health needs of immigrant populations it is essential for those who provide health care not only to know the patterns of disease in the country of origin, but also to avoid unproven assumptions. Social integration is politically and humanely necessary. It does not follow that cultural integration is also necessary or even desirable if it breaks traditional family attitudes and relationships on which mental health may depend. Nor can the wish to integrate or to be integrated be expected to alter any gross differences in metabolic processes. The differences, too, in genetic constitution which produce haemoglobinopathies will remain, although as regards the sickle-cell gene any improvement in standards of living is expected to increase the survival rate of homozygous children, and freedom from malignant malaria will alter the proportions of homozygotes to heterozygotes. Differences of these kinds must be respected, so that special treatment needs are recognized and filled.

Stroud (1971) has stressed the duty of health visitors and other social workers to ensure that immigrant mothers understand medical instructions and are able to carry them out. If the mother has to earn and to work outside the home, the child health centre must arrange times of clinics which she can attend. Health education should be focused on all antenatal women and in the schools special efforts should be made with the girls who are the mothers-to-be. The general practitioner, who is dealing with physical health, should be sharply aware of the vulnerability of immigrant families to anaemia and to vitamin D deficiency. Among the children anaemia may lead to pica and so to lead poisoning (Oppé 1964).

CHAPTER 22

A synthesis

Lord Kelvin is quoted as saying that 'when you could measure what you are speaking about, and express it in numbers, you know something about it'. The intention of this study has been to express in numbers the medical health needs of children in England and Wales from birth to the end of their fifteenth year (0–14 years), derived from existing knowledge of incidence and prevalence of disease and handicap. And the purpose of presenting the amount and the pattern of disease and handicap is to influence the content of paediatric teaching so that doctors can be better prepared for their tasks in caring for children.

CHILD HEALTH NEEDS

Lord Kelvin's claim was limited. Through this numbering you learned 'something', but you did not know the quality of the service required. Hard to measure, this falls into his class of 'knowledge of the meagre and unsatisfactory kind', the fate of knowledge that cannot be 'expressed in numbers'.

Enumeration rests on definition or at least clear description. A definition or a description of child health would be a useful start. Although this difficult intellectual feat is not attempted, some of the fundamental requirements for child health can be identified and not surprisingly they include many non-medical matters. Families are only free to form and develop successfully within a social and political organization in which they are safe from famine, pestilence and war, and under the protection of the law. They need suitable housing and employment, adequate income, opportunity for leisure activities and the child needs appropriate education with preparation for adult life. These requirements will never be adequately met until the family is accorded its proper value by society. Unfortunately in current thinking within the 'modern' mind, the family tends to be denigrated. Well intentioned social legislation, providing support for those who are recognized as unable to attain a 'normal' life unaided, paradoxically acts on those who could as a deterrent to the formation and maintenance of stable family life. As long as social and economic pressures are thoughtlessly mobilized against family life, the health of children will suffer.

All his needs, aimed 'to enable him to develop physically, spiritually and socially in a healthy and normal manner . . . ' are embodied in the 'Declaration of the rights of the child', to which the United Nations assented on 20 November 1959. The tenth and last principle of the declaration ends with the statement of intent that the child shall be brought up 'in full consciousness that his energy and talents should be devoted to the service of his fellow men'. The medical contribution is placed in its true perspective. Governments and politicians, town planning, architects and sanitary engineers, the legal system and those who serve it, all are deeply involved and whatever words are uttered, none of them as yet has made a practical priority of the health of children. This could be due to lack of thought or lack of will as much as to lack of knowledge.

The knowledge comes from medicine and pedagogy supported by psychology, ethology and social science. The medical model builds on disease or deformity, deviations from the normal, and works through therapeutic and investigative efforts to the exposure of cause or causes and so to prevention. While this model serves for adult illness, it neglects one dimension essential for children, the developmental concept. Health is, in one sense, a state of balanced adaptation between the total environment of the child and all his inner drives including his need for physical and intellectual growth towards independence and full maturity. Many factors can upset the balance and this has been recognized in the description of the medical facets of the child health needs described in the first chapter which have to be met by the seven aspects of the practice of paediatrics. One important result of applying the developmental concept has been a movement away from the traditional medicine model based on disease and in the direction of a model based on the promotion of health, the ultimate goal of preventive medicine. Alas! While questions multiply, answers remain few. How can health be promoted? If only even optimal baby feeding programmes were known! The merest glance backwards reveals the swings from starving premature babies to stuffing them, from early addition of solids to late, from governmental provision of one kind of milk to its abandonment as deleterious. Examples of didactic ignorance are too many for the comfort of any doctor engaged to advise about infant feeding. And this is only one area of doubt.

Over the negative promotion of health by the prevention of ill-health there is greater certainty, although even here a prophylaxis which works may not limit its action to the effect desired. The good and proper intention of the therapist affords his patient no protection from side effects, some dangerous to health or even to life itself. Immunization, a public duty no less than a private gain, may produce a neurological deficit without negligence on the part of the doctor, something that society should recognize along with the knowledge that similar disasters can complicate the naturally occurring disease.

These procedures, which require the co-operation of individuals, both doctors and parents, from only a part of the much greater programme to make a safer society for the child. The really large-scale improvements, which, interestingly enough, antedated the discovery of the immediate bacterial and viral cause of epidemics, followed the decade of public health reports that culminated in Edwin Chadwick's 'Report on the sanitary condition of the labouring population of Great Britain' (1842). In the Public Health Act of 1848, government for the first time accepted responsibility for the health of the population and a number of enactments led up to the Public Health Act of 1875. In this Act Government on behalf of society willed an end to the slums. The will survives, but not even now is there a way. A century later a basic minimum standard of housing cannot be ensured within which babies and children can safely grow and develop. Nor are the many methods of accident prevention already recognized fully used.

The safer society depends mainly but not entirely on public health enactments with which the practising physician has little direct concern. It is when, in Charlotte Webb's words, illness is regarded as a public nuisance to be suppressed in the interests of the community, that the personal physician becomes involved. His tasks in relation to improving child health and fulfilling child health needs are twofold. Besides his duties in the treatment of his patient, he can take responsibility for some preventive methods and for advising about the avoidance of risks for the whole child population.

The commitment of society

Viewed against this background, do any practical considerations emerge from the study? The temporal sequence begins with grandparents, their genes and their success in rearing children within a family. That is to say, the family-making skills of parents do relate to their own genetic inheritance and their own childhood experiences. Child health demands 'good' parenting. To what extent this kind of skill can come from precept in the context of education rather than from life's practice at home is difficult to decide.

The family qualifies for a medical-health commitment when the mother becomes pregnant. How does society discharge this commitment?

The chapters into which the Report is divided attempt to enumerate medical health needs in all their great variety. Named and clearly recognizable disease is the easiest to quantify, especially when the patient enters hospital (see Chapter 10). If he dies and the diagnosis is confirmed at autopsy, his medical tabulation is proven and completed. Much medical practice as well as organization aims to prevent or if this be impossible to postpone death. While it is difficult, without appearing callous, not to support the idea that here lies the real business of doctors and of a health service, questions do arise which have to be answered about how far this should be carried and about the proportion of medical and scientific resources that should be so consumed. There are also problems of ethics.

At the other end of the scale comes the promotion of health in so far as knowledge exists of how this may be achieved. The problem can be simplified. Take all possible predictive steps, terminate all pregnancies when there is any risk of abnormality and add euthanasia for good measure for any baby recognized as abnormal who has slipped through the net of prediction. Once more ethical problems arise and the unfortunate prospect that willing human hands with healing as their vocation may not be available to play the role of executioner.

Between these extremes, of allowing men and women and children to die without taking elaborate steps to interfere and of not allowing fetuses to survive or newborn babies to live with any taint of abnormality, lie the confused and sometimes irrational practices now employed, fitted as they are to fallible humanity. Consistency and logic may well be out of place.

Comments from the chapters

The antenatal care of women, safe obstetrics and avoidance of stress or damage to the fetus and the newborn baby prepares him for the optimal care and feeding that should be assured. It is certain that the details as well as the principles of obstetric care insofar as they affect the emotional relationship between mother, father and new baby need to be reviewed. Up-to-date ethological and psychological knowledge has not yet penetrated into this vitally important area, governed still by tradition and routine methods, many of which have long outlived their usefulness. Special care for the newborn should be at least as much a matter of human relationships as it is of scientific apparatus.

Recent thinking about the early months of life has concentrated on screening and assessment, specially of hidden neurological handicaps with a view to early treatment and to minimizing secondary effects both on the child and in the family (see Chapters 3 and 5). Concern with the abnormal has led to some neglect of the main purpose of the first examination which is usually to reassure the parents that the new baby is normal. Surveillance during the first five years may need to be limited to special at-risk groups because of the large case-load that otherwise swamps the health visitor. Families in stressful situations are discussed in Chapter 20. The rate of a child's growth is one indicator of the adequacy of his total care (see Chapter 4).

Towards the end of the first 5-year period, the child's fitness for school and education comes under review and any sensory, motor or perceptual defects which might require special measures must be identified. While the general practitioner with training in appropriate methods should be able to detect abnormalities, a doctor with special experience of school behaviour and of teachers' expectations, methods and outlook has obvious advantages as the adviser on the abnormal child's school management and placement (see Chapter 8). The needs of children with physical and mental handicaps are discussed in Chapters 9 and 13. In both groups much supportive work is required from medically and paediatrically orientated social workers. The basic principles of family acceptance and education in self-care towards the greatest degree of independence apply to both groups of children.

Children with mild mental handicap as well as those with severe mental handicap but without physical defect should be manageable at home. While this is preferable to prolonged stay in institutions, support from doctors, nurses and social workers and available day-care are essential prerequisites. For children with combinations of severe mental and physical handicap, institutional care must be provided. The numbers are large enough to merit special study and special provision, including specialized paediatricians, with co-ordination between the activities of all the professionals in each area.

For families and children with severe emotional disturbances much more expertise is required than present medical training includes (see Chapter 12). Lectures is psychology and in the normal course of emotional development in the human should form part of pre-clinical education along with anatomy and physiology. The teaching of psycho-paediatrics and practical experience in counselling and in methods of handling disturbed children and their families are essential for all doctors who will have responsibility, be it medical or surgical, for the treatment of children.

The necessity for teamwork is described in Chapter 1 and again in relation to children with spina bifida and to children in depriving and abusing families. Although everyone acknowledges this need, co-operation, co-ordination of effort and sharing of information still present great practical difficulties. Too much clamour for teamwork, with the innuendo that this or that person is not competent to tackle the problem, can produce the bitter resistance born of professional pride or vicious inter-professional conflict over status. In the training of all personnel, medical as well as of allied professions, more attention should be paid to the recognition of these natural human reactions. The difficulties will not be resolved until those who have to work together understand and respect each other's knowledge and function. It is for the leaders and the teachers to set the example.

Certain important and relatively common medical conditions are discussed in Chapters 16, 17 and 18. These might well be chapters in a text book of paediatrics the accent being on management and those aspects of treatment other than by drugs and operations. Quantification shows what is common and what is rare and could guide the programme of teaching and training at general and vocational levels.

Attention is drawn in Chapter 11 to the differences between hospital and general practice. The greater degree of organization of general practice with increasing opportunities for research and study will undoubtedly attract many of the students who would in earlier days have attempted to climb the hospital ladder in order to practice general medicine. The specialization now necessary for advancement in hospital medicine will force more of the teaching out of hospital and into the community. As far as paediatrics is concerned this considerable re-orientation will be welcomed.

In Chapter 19 the prevalence of accidents is discussed in some detail. More steps are urgently required in the prevention of home accidents. As regards Accident and Emergency Departments special arrangements for segregation of children are not yet in full operation. It should not be necessary to observe that the standard of treatment is not affected merely by changing the name on the door from Casualty to Accident and Emergency department. Direct participation in the work by paediatricians, psychiatrists and epidemiologists together with social workers is essential if the damaging long-term effects of accidents are to be controlled and repeated accidents avoided.

The Report concluded

The original terms of reference for the joint working party were to give further consideration 'to the role of the general practitioner, the health authority medical officer, the health visitor and the district nurse'. The working party took the view that the first step would have to be to mobilize and to make accessible all the available data on the quantity of the different kinds of medical service required by children.

That study, now completed, is presented in the Report. Two results could follow. The first would be to make possible a realistic teaching programme in elementary paediatrics directed to the common happenings in childhood to be used in the training of all who are concerned or likely to be concerned with child health. The second would be to attempt to dispose of trained personnel in the most appropriate ways. Since 1968 the British Paediatric Association has published its own view of 'Paediatrics in the seventies' and the Department of Health has set up a Committee under the chairmanship of Dr Donald Court with the task of co-ordinating the labours of those working in 'child health'. Thus the working party was relieved of the second of its functions and for the most part, service plans have been purposely excluded from the discussion.

In 1971 the American Academy of Paediatrics published the results of a 3-year study of child health care orientated towards its availability, its quality and especially its delivery. This, which is difficult enough here, presents a much more difficult problem for a nation lacking a National Health Service. It was the title of this Report, 'Lengthening Shadows', that prompted the Director to 'Widening Horizons'. As children grow, their shadows do truly lengthen, but shadows are sad, dark, depressing things, longest in the evening and shortest when the day is at its brightest and the sun is highest in the heavens. Shadows, however long or short, have overtones of sadness, even of pessimism. By contrast the country which has placed some of its sons upon the moon, has given to men, both metaphorically and literally, their widest horizons yet.

From the vantage point of present knowledge, we can see much of what needs doing to give to all our children the chance to develop their potential to the full in the context of a strong and happy family life. As supply always creates demand social and medical work have to be conducted permanently within the framework of scarcity, and that means a system of priorities, priorities which must be planned by doctors. It also requires administrative excellence, and the recognition by administrators of their two main functions. These are first, to provide the environment in which professionals can best work in meeting the basic needs of the health of the population and, second, on behalf of the patient, to secure a line of minimum standards everywhere, below which the service will not be permitted to operate. What is good can be distributed to all, but not what is best.

There is always a danger that neat administration will itself become the objective of a health service rather than the provision of service. It will indeed be a bad day for medicine if ever its practitioners are compelled to replace their symbol, the serpent of Aesculapius, with the bed of Procrustes.

What is known about the medical needs of children has been gathered into this Report. The task is described. To perform it the real lack may not be manpower nor money so much as the rational use of what is available. And this demands above all the will to use it in making a true and absolute priority of this great aim – the health of children.

Appendices

APPENDIX I

Two definitions

Incidence is the inception rate of new cases.

Prevalence is the rate, in a population, of existing cases and depends upon the incidence modified by the duration of the condition and its mortality rate.

APPENDIX II

Home populations as at 30 June 1971 (from RGSR)

All ages, total	M	23 797 500	48 894 500
	F	25 097 000	
School children (5–15)	M	3 980 100	7 756 600
	F	3 776 500	
Under 5	M	2 009 100	3 919 900
	F	1 910 800	
Under 1	M	401 500	781 600
	F	380 100	
Live births (1971)	M	403 223	783 155
	F	379 932	
School entrants 1971	M	410 200	800 600
	F	390 400	
All ages under 15 years	M	5 989 200	11 676 500
	F	5 687 300	

APPENDIX III

Estimated total child populations by sex and age as at 30 June 1971 (from RGSR 1971 Table 1) (in thousands)

Age		*Persons*	*Males*	*Females*
0–		781.6	401.5	380.1
1–		754.2	386.4	367.8
2–		795.9	407.5	388.4
3–		787.6	403.5	384.1
4–		800.6	410.2	390.4
	Total	3 919.9	2 009.1	1 910.8
5–		812.3	416.9	395.4
6–		823.2	421.5	401.7
7–		829.2	425.8	403.4
8–		816.5	417.5	399.0
9–		801.8	411.0	390.8
	Total	4 083.0	2 092.7	1 990.3
10–		771.8	396.5	375.3
11–		749.5	384.6	364.9
12–		732.6	376.7	355.9
13–		721.1	370.1	351.0
14–		698.6	359.5	339.1
	Total	3 673.6	1 887.4	1 786.2
All under 15–		11 676.5	5 989.2	5 687.3
All under 18–		13 703.7	7 032.1	6 671.6
Total population		48 894.5	23 797.5	25 097.0
Live births				
Legitimate		717.477	369.262	348.215
Illegitimate		65.678	33.961	31.717
	Total	783.155	403.223	379.932

Still births	9 899
Neonatal deaths (under 4 weeks)	9 113

Perinatal mortality rate: 22 per 1 000

Deaths in the first year: 13 720

Death rate in first year: 18 per 1 000 live births

APPENDIX IV

Estimated home populations, by sex and age, as at 30 June 1971 in hospital regions (from RGSR Table 2) (in thousands)

Hospital regions		*All ages*	*Under 1 year*	*1–4 years*	*5–9 years*	*10–14 years*	*Total 0–14 years*
Newcastle	M	1489.7	25.1	100.5	136.5	130.4	766.5
	F	1557.4	23.8	96.1	130.0	124.1	
Leeds	M	1564.2	27.3	107.1	138.9	128.5	783.0
	F	1667.8	25.8	103.2	131.9	119.8	
Sheffield	M	2295.8	39.8	161.6	205.0	184.1	1152.5
	F	2357.9	37.7	153.7	195.9	174.7	
East Anglia	M	868.7	14.1	57.6	74.1	66.3	413.6
	F	894.0	13.3	55.4	70.4	62.4	
N.W. Met.	M	2066.4	34.3	127.3	170.7	152.0	945.3
	F	2186.5	32.6	121.1	162.0	145.3	
N.E. Met.	M	1589.1	27.0	107.1	137.6	123.2	769.5
	F	1679.8	25.6	101.5	131.2	116.4	
S.E. Met.	M	1628.6	26.1	107.1	140.4	125.3	770.6
	F	1800.4	24.7	101.5	132.8	118.7	
S.W. Met.	M	1567.5	24.9	94.5	128.2	114.9	709.4
	F	1732.8	23.6	90.5	122.7	110.1	
Wessex	M	990.2	16.1	68.7	86.7	77.2	516.2
	F	1064.2	15.2	63.5	83.1	74.1	
Oxford	M	992.0	17.6	73.5	93.7	81.4	516.9
	F	1007.6	16.6	69.9	88.9	76.1	
South Western	M	1528.8	24.2	99.4	129.7	119.0	722.6
	F	1648.0	20.7	94.4	122.9	112.3	
Welsh	M	1324.5	21.9	88.6	116.4	107.2	651.9
	F	1400.7	20.7	84.9	110.5	101.7	
Birmingham	M	2533.1	45.3	183.1	229.6	204.2	1288.7
	F	2585.6	42.8	174.3	218.6	190.8	
Manchester	M	2207.3	38.4	155.4	199.0	176.6	1110.1
	F	2336.8	36.4	147.5	188.9	167.9	
Liverpool	M	1073.7	19.4	77.6	106.2	97.1	584.1
	F	1145.9	18.3	73.2	100.5	91.8	

APPENDIX V

Death by cause – sex and age group, 1971 (from RGSR Table 17)

Annual deaths		*Days* 0	*Days* 1–6	*Weeks* 1	*Weeks* 2	*Weeks* 3	*Months* 1–2	*Months* 3–5	*Months* 6–8	*Months* 9–11	*Years* 0	*Years* 1	*Years* 2	*Years* 3	*Years* 4	*Years* 0–4	*Years* 5–9	*Years* 10–14	*Total*	*Percentage of total deaths*
I. Infective and	M	3	26	20	11	15	97	75	49	29	325	35	15	8	5	388	30	10	805	4.34
parasitic	F	3	12	18	12	6	77	66	24	20	238	51	29	13	12	343	21	13		
II. Neoplastic	M	2	2	1	2	1	7	5	4	8	32	33	39	33	35	172	169	124	837	4.52
	F	6	2	2	—	1	6	3	12	2	34	26	23	37	22	142	139	91		
III. Endocrine nutri-	M	3	11	12	1	2	19	20	6	8	80	10	4	5	6	105	35	19	272	1.46
tional and metabolic	F	2	8	1	3	—	11	11	7	5	48	10	3	8	6	75	25	13		
IV. Blood and blood	M	1	2	1	—	—	2	—	—	1	7	4	—	—	3	14	13	3	56	0.30
forming organs	F	—	1	2	1	—	1	1	1	2	9	2	2	4	2	19	3	4		
V. Mental disorders	M	—	—	—	—	—	—	—	—	—	—	3	1	—	2	6	1	—	14	0.07
	F	—	—	—	—	—	—	—	—	—	—	1	—	—	1	2	2	3		
VI. Disease of nervous	M	—	14	17	14	6	31	27	20	16	145	31	16	14	14	220	46	43	534	2.88
system and sense organs	F	1	10	14	4	5	28	28	12	12	114	21	20	8	6	169	34	22		
VII. Circulatory system	M	—	—	3	1	—	17	7	8	5	41	12	9	1	3	66	22	27	204	1.10
	F	—	7	2	—	1	7	7	5	2	31	9	6	1	4	51	12	26		
VIII. Respiratory	M	26	70	52	51	50	527	428	131	65	1 400	102	56	36	18	1 612	71	48	3 060	16.52
system	F	15	52	31	34	30	361	308	130	67	1 028	90	52	33	22	1 225	57	47		
IX. Digestive system	M	48	30	12	6	5	19	27	4	3	156	10	7	4	5	182	17	13	368	1.98
	F	46	22	9	3	4	15	16	4	4	123	6	4	4	1	138	12	6		
X. Genito-urinary	M	2	2	4	3	2	10	8	1	1	33	3	3	2	3	44	14	10	108	0.58
system	F	—	—	—	—	1	4	4	1	—	10	3	2	1	1	17	9	14		
XI. Complications of	M	—	—	—	—	—	—	—	—	—	—	—	—	—	—	—	—	—	1	0.00
pregnancy etc.	F	—	—	—	—	—	—	—	—	—	—	—	—	—	—	—	—	1		
XII. Skin and	M	—	2	—	—	—	—	1	—	1	4	1	—	—	—	5	—	—	11	0.06
subcutaneous tissues	F	—	—	—	—	—	1	3	—	—	4	1	—	—	1	6	—	—		

Annual deaths		Days		Weeks			Months				Years					Years			Total	Percentage of total deaths
		0	1–6	1	2	3	1–2	3–5	6–8	9–11	0	1	2	3	4	0–4	5–9	10–14		
XIII. Musculo-skeletal	M	—	—	—	—	—	—	—	—	—	—	1	—	1	2	4	2	2	16	0.08
and connective tissue	F	—	1	—	—	—	—	—	1	—	2	—	—	—	1	3	4	1		
XIV. Congenital	M	405	382	166	67	72	264	124	72	42	1 594	92	47	36	34	1 803	94	66	3 627	19.58
anomalies	F	311	301	164	73	56	209	142	56	44	1 356	103	34	24	25	1 542	76	46		
XV. Perinatal morbidity	M	2 275	1 303	88	24	15	19	5	—	2	3 731	1	—	—	—	3 732	—	—	6 161	33.27
and mortality	F	1 505	788	79	16	12	21	5	2	—	2 428	1	—	—	—	2 429	—	—		
XVI. Ill-defined	M	2	1	4	3	7	86	60	8	7	178	5	3	—	1	187	3	2	320	1.72
conditions	F	—	3	1	2	2	48	47	9	6	118	6	—	—	1	125	3	—		
XVII. Accidents,	M	9	10	7	4	5	79	74	32	28	248	107	124	95	88	662	399	323	2 122	11.46
poisoning and violence	F	15	8	10	1	9	56	52	24	28	203	69	59	63	42	436	171	131		
All causes	M	2 776	1 855	387	187	180	1 177	861	335	216	7 974	450	324	235	219	9 202	916	690		
	F	1 904	1 215	333	149	127	845	693	288	192	5 746	399	234	196	147	6 722	568	418		
		4 680	3 070	720	336	307	2 022	1 554	623	408	13 720	849	558	431	366	15 924	1 484	1 108	18 516	99.92

APPENDIX VI

Deaths classified by certain external causes (from RGSR 1971 Table 17)

	Under 2 years	*0–4*	*5–14*	*Total*	
EXVII Accident, poisoning, violence ICD 800–999	623	1096	1024	2122	
Traffic accident					
Railway 800–807	1	5	11	16	
Motor vehicle 810–819	41	245	574	819	Road traffic (1) **836**
Connected with motor vehicle 820–827	4	5	12	17	
Water transport 830–838	0	2	18	20	
Air transport 840–845	0	0	0	0	
Accidental poisoning					
Drugs 850–859	7	17	5	22	
Other solid substances 860–869	4	6	1	7	
Gases 870–877	5 (CO=3)	6	11	17	
Falls 880–887	38	68	67	**135**	Falls (7)
Fire and flames 890–899	37	97	41	**138**	Fire and flames (5)
Environmental 900–909	31	32	4	36	
Suicide 950–959	0	0	4	4	
Homicide 960–969	52 (38 0–1)	68	29	97	Non-accidental injury (6) **137**
Possible homicide 980–989	peak at 3–5 mos. 20 (16 0–1)	28	12	40	
Other 910–929	383	514	232	746	
Drowning 910	26	103	127	**230**	Drowning (3)
Respiratory obstruction					Suffocation e.g.
Food 911	207 (190 0–1)	224	9	**233**	food (2)
Other 912	9	13	3	16	
Suffocation 913	114 (99 0–1)	125	24	**149**	Mechanical suffocation (4)

The 13 per cent of the child population below the age of 2 years provided 29.4 per cent of total deaths.
The order of frequency of the main external causes of death is shown in brackets on the right-hand side of the table.

APPENDIX VII

Injuries : estimated total discharges and deaths
Taken from HIPE 1971 (Table 5) and number of deaths taken from RGSR 1971 (Tables 17 and 18D) classified by nature of injury

Nature of injury ICD	*0–4*	*5–14*	*Total*	*Total Deaths*	*Traffic Accident Deaths*	*Deaths from Falls*
Fractures						
involving skull 800–804	2 990	4 263	7 253	547	264	83
and dislocations 805–809	110	975	1 085	98	4	0
single and multiple 810–829	5 094	17 639	22 733	14	68	7
Dislocations 830–839	133	1 096	1 229	11	9	1
Sprains and Strains 840–848	110	565	675	0	0	0
Concussion 850	2 846	6 666	9 512	8	0	0
Brain injury 851–854	14 273	22 843	37 116	192	77	30
Visceral injury 860–869	166	963	1 129	238	131	13
Wound of eye 870–871	409	919	1 328	0	0	0
Wound of ear 872	55	22	77	0	0	0
Laceration of head 873	1 495	1 760	3 255	1	0	0
Open wounds 874–907	1 362	4 440	5 802	14	0	0
Superficial injury 910–918	443	1 207	1 650	0	0	1
Contusions 920–929	1 339	3 278	4 617	2	0	0
Nerve injuries 950–959	33	266	299	3	0	0
Foreign body 930–939	2 846	1 782	4 628	253		
Burns 940–949	4 650	2 126	6 776	60		
Adverse effects of drugs 960–979	16 742	2 536	19 278	27		
Toxic effect 980–989	8 748	1 251	9 999	131		
Physical agents 990–996	1 461	2 724	4 185	514		
Others 997–999	1 262	2 336	3 598	3		
Total	66 567	79 657	146 224	2 122	553	135

APPENDIX VIII

Estimated total discharges and deaths by ICD categories (from HIPE 1971 Table 5) and number of deaths (from RGSR 1971 Table 17)

ICD 960–967. XVII Adverse effects of medicinal and non-medicinal substances	*0–4*	*5–14*	*Total*	*RGSR deaths Table 17*
Medicinal substances				
Antibiotics	255	55	310	0
Other anti-infectives	188	22	210	1
Hormones	343	33	376	0
Primarily systemic agents	299	22	321	2
Agents affecting blood	897	33	930	1
Analgesics and antipyretics	7 231	741	7 972	9
Anticonvulsants	177	44	221	0
Other sedatives	875	255	1 130	0
CNS depressants	11	0	11	0
Local anaesthetics	199	11	210	0
Psychotherapeutic agents	1 749	576	2 325	5
CNS stimulants	77	22	99	0
Agents primarily affecting :				
Autonomic nervous system	886	55	941	3
Cardiovascular system	244	22	266	3
Gastro-intestinal system	244	22	266	0
Diuretics	44	22	66	0
Other unspecified drugs	2 979	587	3 566	1
Two or more medicines	44	11	55	1
Alcohol with specified medicine	0	0	0	0
Non-medicinal substances				
Alcohol	277	177	454	0
Petroleum products	1 340	44	1 384	1
Industrial solvents	1 539	55	1 594	0
Corrosives, acids, alkalis	1 473	155	1 628	3
Lead and compounds	33	11	44	2
Other metals	77	11	88	0
Carbon monoxide	11	11	22	120
Other gases, vapours, fumes	122	55	177	1
Noxious foodstuffs	1 262	542	1 804	0
Other non-medicinal substances	2 613	188	2 801	2
Other external causes	276	410	686	510
Early complications of trauma	0	110	110	0
Injury, other and unspecified causes	1 174	2 192	3 366	5
Others	1 262	2 447	3 709	5
Total	28 201	8 941	37 032	675

APPENDIX IX

Estimated total discharges and deaths
Taken from HIPE (Tables 20ii and 19ii – 1971) classified by nature of injury

ICD D list	*Home accidents*				*Road traffic accidents*		
	Under 1 year	*0–4*	*5–14*	*Total*	*0–4*	*5–14*	*Total*
Fractures of skull, spine and trunk N800–809	580	1 360	390	1 750	510	1 710	2 220
Limbs N810–829	260	1 740	2 320	4 060	980	2 920	3 900
Dislocations, sprains without fracture N830–845	0	50	150	200	10	70	80
Intracranial injury without skull fracture N850–854	1 420	7 470	3 890	11 360	2 310	7 380	9 690
Internal injury N860–869	0	40	30	70	80	370	450
Lacerations, superficial injuries and contusions N870–929	130	1 930	2 280	4 210	520	1 800	2 320
Foreign body entering through orifice N930–939	160	780	410	1 190	20	0	20
Burns N940–949	570	3 350	1 020	4 370	10	10	20
Injury to nerves spinal cord N950–959	0	0	20	20	10	0	10
Adverse effect of medicinal agent N960–979	200	6 180	580	6 760	10	0	10
Non-medicinal toxic substance N980–989	300	3 550	250	3 800	0	0	0
Other N990–996	70	520	470	990	20	280	300
All injuries	3 710	27 090	11 840	38 930	4 500	14 550	19 050
All injuries at all ages				99 370			92 190

Children under 15 provide 39 per cent of all home accidents and 20.6 per cent of road traffic accidents treated in hospital.

References

Ack, M., Muller, I. & Weil, W. B. (1961). Intelligence of children with diabetes mellitus. *Pediatrics,* 28, 764–70.

Alberman, E. D., Butler, N. R. & Gardiner, P. A. (1971). Children with squint at seven years: a handicapped group? *Practitioner,* 206, 501–6.

Alberman, E. D. & Goldstein, H. (1970). The 'at risk' register: a statistical evaluation. *Brit. J. prev. Soc. Med.,* 24, 129–35.

Andrews, G. & Harris, M. (1964). *The syndrome of stuttering.* Clinics in develop. Med., No. 14. Heinemann, London.

Andry, N. (1741). *L'orthopédie ou l'art de prévenir et de corriger dans les enfants les difformités du corps.* Alix, Lambert & Durand, Paris.

Ansell, B. (1975). Personal communication.

Arneil, G. C. & Crosbie, J. C. (1963). Infantile rickets returns to Glasgow. *Lancet,* 1, 423–5.

Arthurton, M. W. (1972). Immigrant children and the day-to-day work of a paediatrician. *Arch. Dis. Childh.,* 47, 126.

Asher, P. & Schonell, F. E. (1950). A survey of 400 cases of cerebral palsy in childhood. *Arch. Dis. Childh.,* 25, 360–79.

Barlow, T. G. (1966). Congenital dislocation of the hip in the newborn. *Proc. roy. Soc. Med.,* 59, 1, 103.

Barltrop, D. (1971). Lead poisoning. *Arch. Dis. Childh.,* 46, 233–5.

Barltrop, D. & Killala, N. J. P. (1969). Factors influencing exposure of children to lead. *Ibid.,* 44, 476–9.

Beals, R. K. (1969). Homocystinuria. *J. Bone Jt. Surg.,* 51A, 1564–72.

Benson, P. F. Stroud, C. E., Mitchell, N. J. & Nicolaides, A. (1963). Rickets in immigrant children in London. *Brit. med. J.,* 1, 1054–6.

Beutler, E. & Baluda, M. C. (1966). A simple spot screening test for galactosemia. *J. Lab. Clin. Med.,* 68, 137–41.

Beutler, E., Baluda, M. C., Sturgeon, P. & Day, R. (1965). A new genetic abnormality resulting in galactose-1-phosphate uridyltransferase deficiency. *Lancet,* 1, 353–4

Biggs, R. (1976). Personal communication.

Bignell, J. R. (1971). Tuberculosis in England and Wales in the next 20 years. *Post-grad. med. J.,* 47, 759–62.

Bloom, A., Hayes, T. M. & Gamble, D. R. (1975). Register of newly diagnosed diabetic children. *Brit. med. J.,* 3, 580–3.

Bobath, K. (1966). The motor deficits in patients with cerebral palsy. *Clinics in Develop. Med.,* No. 23. Heinemann, London.

Bowlby, J. (1951). *Maternal care and mental health.* WHO Monograph No. 2. Geneva.

Bransby, E. R., Curley, G. & Kotulanska, M. (1973). A study of patients notified by hospitals as addicted to drugs. Second report. *Health Trends,* 5, 17–20.

Britten, M. I., Spooner, R. J. D., Dormandy, K. M. & Biggs, R. (1966). The haemophilic boy in school. *Brit. med. J.* 2, 224.

Brock, D. J. H. & Sutcliffe, R. G. (1972). Alpha-fetoprotein in the antenatal diagnosis of anencephaly and spina bifida. *Lancet,* 2, 197.

Bronks, I. G. & Blackburn, E. K. (1968). A socio-medical study of haemophilia and related states. *Brit. J. prev. soc. Med.,* 22, 68–72.

Brubaker, R. F., Wong, V. G., Schulman, J. D., Seegmiller, J. E. & Kuwabara, T. (1970). Benign cystinosis. *Amer. J. Med.*, 49, 546–50.

Bruch, H. (1939). Physical growth and development of obese children. *Amer. J. Dis. Child.*, 58, 457.

Bruch, H. (1939). Basal metabolism and serum cholesterol of obese children. *Loc. cit*, 100.

Bruch, H. (1940). Physiological and psychologic aspects of the food intake of obese children. *Ibid.*, 59, 739.

Butterfield, W. J. H. (1968). *Priorities in medicine.* Nuffield Provincial Hospital Trust. pp. 14–15.

Cancer (1971). Report of the standing sub-committee on Cancer. *Central Health Services Council Report for the year 1970*, Appendix III. HMSO, London.

Catterall, A. (1971). The natural history of Perthes' disease. *J. Bone Jt. Surg.*, 53B, 37–53.

Cohen, Sir H. (1956). *Report of the sub-committee on the medical care of epileptics.* HMSO, London.

Colliss, V. R. (1972). The effects of selective treatment of myelomeningocele on a neonatal unit. *Develop. Med. Child Neurol.*, 14, 24–37, Supp. 27.

Council of Europe (1972). *Mass screening and possibility of treatment and/or the prevention of certain hereditary enzymopathies and proteinopathies presenting clinical consequences.* Strasbourg.

Court, D. & Jackson, A. (1972). *Paediatrics in the seventies.* OUP.

Curtis Jenkins, G. H. (1973). Personal communication.

Davie, R., Butler, N. & Goldstein, H. (1972). *From birth to seven.* Longman (NCB), London, p. 90.

Dawson, B., Horobin, G., Illsley, R. & Mitchell, R. (1967). A survey of childhood asthma in Aberdeen. *Lancet,* 1, 827–30.

de Dombal, F. T., Horrocks, J. C., Walmsley, G. & Wilson, P. D. (1975). Computer-aided diagnosis and decision-making in the acute abdomen. *J. roy. Coll. Phycns. Lond.*, 9, 211–18.

DHSS (1971). *Census of children in non-psychiatric hospitals in England and Wales on 7 October 1970.* DHSS, London.

Douglas, J. W. B. (1964). *The home and the school.* MacGibbon & Kee, London.

Douglas, J. W. B. & Bloomfield, J. M. (1958). *Children under five.* London.

Douglas, J. W. B., Ross, J. M. & Simpson, H. R. (1968). *All our future.* Peter Davies, London.

Dubowitz, V. (1965). Intellectual impairment in muscular dystrophy. *Arch. Dis. Childh.*, 40, 296–301.

Dubowitz, V. (1973). Personal communication.

Dudgeon, J. A. (1975). Personal communication.

Eid, E. E. (1970). Follow-up study of children having excessive weight gain in first six months of life. *Brit. med. J.*, 2, 74–76.

Etzwiler, D. D. (1962). What the juvenile diabetic knows about his disease. *Pediatrics,* 29, 135–41.

Etzwiler, D. D. (1967). Who's teaching the diabetic? *Diabetes,* 16, 111–17.

Etzwiler, D. D. & Sines, L. K. (1962). Juvenile diabetes and its management: family, social, and academic implications. *J. Amer. med. Ass.*, 181, 304–8.

Fine, S. (1968). *Blind and partially sighted children.* DSE Education Survey No. 4. HMSO, London.

Finer, Sir M. (1974). *Report of the committee on one-parent families.* HMSO, London.

Finlay, H. V. L., Maudsley, R. H. & Busfield, P. I. (1967). Dislocatable and dislocated hip in the newborn infant. *Brit. med. J.*, 4, 377–81.

Fitz, R. H. (1886). Perforating inflammation of the vermiform appendix, with

special reference to its early diagnosis and treatment. *Trans. Ass. Amer. Phscn.,* 1, 107–35.
Franklin, A. W. (1960). 'There is nothing the matter with your child'. *Practitioner,* 185, 64–70.
Friedland, J., Perle, G., Saifer, A., Schneck, L. & Volk, B. W. (1971). Screening for Tay-Sachs disease in utero using amniotic fluid. *Proc. soc. Exp. Biol. Med.,* 136, 1297–8.
Froggatt, P., Lynas, M. A. & MacKenzie, G. (1971). Epidemiology of sudden unexpected death in infants ('cot death') in Northern Ireland. *Brit. J. prev. Soc. Med.,* 25, 119.
Fuller, A. (1973). Personal communication.
Gardner, P. S., Turk, D. C., Ahern, W. A., Bird, T., Holdaway, M. D. & Court, S. D. M. (1967). Deaths associated with respiratory tract infection in childhood. *Brit. med. J.,* 4, 316–20.
Gastaut, H. (1965). *Enquiry into the education of epileptic children.* Epilepsy and education seminar in Marseilles, 1964. British Epilepsy Association and International Association for Epilepsy, 1965.
George, L. & Norman, A. P. (1971). Life tables for cystic fibrosis. *Arch. Dis. Childh.,* 46, 139–43.
Glucksman, M. L. (1972). Psychiatric observations on obesity. In Reichsman, F. (1972).
Goldman, H., Scriver, C. & Aaron, K. (1970). Use of dithriothreitol to correct cystine storage in cultured cystinotic fibroblasts. *Lancet,* 1, 811–12.
Gough, C. W. (1954). *Legge-Calvé-Perthes syndrome.* Thomas, Baltimore.
G. P. Survey (1960). A survey of the epilepsies in general practice. *Brit. med. J.,* 2, 416.
Greenwood, M. (1948). *Medical statistics from Graunt to Farr.* Cambridge.
Griffiths, M. I. & Barrett, N. M. (1967). Cerebral palsy in Birmingham. *Develop. Med. Child Neurol.,* 9, 33–46.
Hall, M. H. (1975). In *Concerning child abuse,* ed. A. W. Franklin, Churchill Livingstone, Edinburgh, London & New York.
Hansen, E. (1960). Cerebral palsy in Denmark. *Acta psychiat.* (Kbh), 35, supp. 146.
Hay, J. D. (1966). Population and clinic studies of congenital heart disease in Liverpool. *Brit. med. J.,* 2, 661.
Heald, F. P. (1972). The natural history of obesity. P. 104. In Reichsman, F. (1972).
Henderson, J. L. (1961). Ed. *Cerebral palsy in childhood and adolescence.* Livingstone, Edinburgh & London.
Hernberg, S. & Nikkanen, J. (1970). Enzyme inhibition by lead under normal urban conditions. *Lancet,* 1, 63.
Higgins, I. T. (1965). The epidemiology of congenital heart disease. *J. chron. Dis.,* 18, 699–721.
Hill, Sir J. D. N. (1968). *Hospital treatment of acute poisoning: report of the joint sub-committee.* HMSO, London.
Holmes, A. M., Enoch, B. A., Taylor, J. L. & Jones, M. E. (1973). Occult rickets and osteomalacia amongst the Asian immigrant population. *Quart. J. med.,* n.s. 42, 125–49.
House of Lords (1970). Debate 28 February reported. *Lancet,* 1, 481.
Howells, J. G. (1972). *Family psychiatry for child psychiatrists.* Society of clinical psychiatrists special report.
Hubble, D. (1969). Ed. Paediatric endocrinology (chapter 9 by J. K. Lloyd & O. H. Wolff). Blackwell, Oxford & Edinburgh.
Huntsman, R. G., Lehmann, H. (1974). Treatment of sickle-cell disease. *Brit. J. Haematol.,* 28, 437–44.

Husband, P. & Hinton, P. E. (1972). Families of children with repeated accidents. *Arch. Dis. Childh.,* 47, 396–400.

Ingram, T. T. S. (1964). Paediatric aspects of cerebral palsy. Livingstone, Edinburgh & London.

Jackson, G. (1972). Child abuse syndrome: the cases we miss. *Brit. med. J.,* 3, 756–7.

James, J. I. P. (1967). *Scoliosis.* Livingstone, Edinburgh.

Kamhi, E. & MacEwen, G. D. (1975). Treatment of Legge-Calvé-Perthes Disease: prognostic value of Catterall's classification. *J. Bone Jt. Surg.,* 57A, 651–4.

Kattamis, C., Touliatos, N., Haidus, S. & Matsaniotis, N. (1970). Growth of children with thalassaemia. *Arch. Dis. Childh.,* 45, 502.

Kessel, N. (1965). Self-poisoning. *Brit. med. J.,* 2, 1265.

Knox, E. G. & Mahon, D. F. (1970). Evaluation of 'infant at risk' registers. *Arch. Dis. Childh.,* 45, 634–9.

Kolvin, I., Mac Keith, R. C. & Meadow, S. R. (1973). *Bladder control and enuresis.* Clinics in Developmental Medicine, Nos. 48/49. Heinemann, London.

Komrower, G. (1976). Personal communication.

Krieger, I. & Mellinger, R. C. (1971). Pituitary function in the deprivation syndrome, *J. Pediat.,* 79, 216.

Kushlick, A. (1968). Social problems of mental subnormality. In *Foundations of child psychiatry,* ed. E. Miller. Pergamon, Oxford & London.

Kushlick, A. (1972). Personal communication.

Lack, I. (1964). Examination of the incidence of malformations for evidence of drug teratogenesis. *Brit. J. prev. Soc. Med.,* 18, 196–201.

Lane, J. M. & Millar, J. D. (1969). Routine childhood vaccination against smallpox reconsidered. *New Engl. J. Med.,* 281, 1220.

Langford, W. S., Gilder, R., Wilking, V. N., Genn, M. M. & Sherrill, H. H. (1953). Pilot study of childhood accidents: preliminary report. *Pediatrics,* 11, 405.

Lansdowne, Marquis of (1927). *The Petty Papers.* Constable, London.

Laurence, K. M. (1966). The survival of untreated spina bifida cystica. *Develop. Med. Child Neurol.* supp. 11.

Levy, H. L., Madigan, P. M. & Peneva, P. (1971). Evidence for delayed histidine transamination in neonates with histidinemia. *Pediatrics,* 47, 128.

Levy, H. L. (1974). Genetic screening. In *Advances in Human Genetics,* Vol. IV, Plenum Press, New York.

Linde, L. M., Rasof, B., Dunn, O. J. & Robb, E. (1966). Attitudinal factors in congenital heart disease. *Pediatrics,* 38, 92–101.

Livingston, S. (1963). *Living with epileptic seizures.* Thomas, Springfield.

Lloyd, J. K., Wolff, O. H. & Whalen, W. S. (1961). Childhood obesity: a long-term study of height and weight. *Brit. med. J.,* 2, 145–48.

Lorber, J. (1971). Results of treatment of myelomeningocele. *Develop. Med. Child Neurol.,* 13, 279–303.

Lotter, V. (1966). Epidemiology of autistic conditions in young children. *Soc. Psychiat.,* 1, 124.

McGregor, R. M. (1969). *The work of a family doctor.* Livingstone, Edinburgh & London.

Mac Keith, R. C. (1975). In *Concerning child abuse,* ed. A. W. Franklin. Churchill Livingstone, Edinburgh, London & New York.

Mac Keith, R. & Rutter, M. (1972). A note on the prevalence of language disorders in young children. In *The child with delayed speech,* ed. M. Rutter & J. A. M. Martin. Clinics in Develop. Med., No. 43. Heinemann, London.

McKeown, T. & Record, R. G. (1960). Malformations in a population observed for five years after birth. In *Ciba Foundation Symposium on Congenital Malformations,* ed. G. E. W. Wolstenholme & C. M. O'Connor. Churchill, London, 2–16.

McKeown, T. & Teruel, J. R. (1970). An assessment of the feasibility of discharge of patients in hospitals for the subnormal. *Brit. J. prev. Soc. Med.,* 24, 116–19.

McNicol, M. W., Mikhail, J. R. & Sutherland, I. (1971). Tuberculosis in Brent. *Post-grad. med. J.* 47, 691–3.

Manson, M. M., Logan, W. P. D. & Loy, R. M. (1960). *Rubella and other virus infections during pregnancy.* Min. Hlth. Reports on Medical Subjects No. 101. London.

Martin, H. L. (1970). Antecedents of burns and scalds in children. *Brit J. med. Psychol.,* 43, 39.

Mason Brown, J. J. (1956). Acute appendicitis in infancy and childhood. *J. roy. Coll. Surg. Edin.,* 1, 268–84.

Matthew, H. (1972–3). Drug overdose. In *Poisoning and drug induced disease.* Medicine No. 4, ed. S. Campbell-Smith.

Meadow, S. R., White, R. H. R. & Johnston, N. M. (1969). Prevalence of symptomless urinary tract disease in Birmingham schoolchildren. Pyuria and bacteriuria. *Brit. med. J.,* 3, 81.

Menkes, J. H., Andrews, J. M. & Cancilla, P. A. (1971). The cerebroretinal degenerations. *J. Pediat.,* 79, 183–96.

Meyer, R. J. & Klein, D. (1969). Childhood injuries (ed.). *Pediatrics,* 44, 791–896.

Millar, J. A., Cumming, R. L. C., Battistini, V., Carswell, F. & Goldberg, A. (1970). Lead and delta-aminolaevulinic acid dehydratase levels in mentally retarded children and in lead-poisoned suckling rats. *Lancet,* 2, 695–8.

Miller, F. J. W., Court, S. D. M., Knox, E. G., Brandon, S. (1974). *The school years in Newcastle upon Tyne,* Oxford University Press.

Miller, F. J. W., Court, S. D. M., Walton, W. S. & Knox, E. G. (1960). *Growing up in Newcastle upon Tyne.* Oxford University Press.

Millichap, J. G. (1968). *Febrile convulsions.* Macmillan, New York.

Ministry of Health (1965). Enquiry into sudden death in infancy. Special Report No. 113. HMSO, London.

Morton, T. G. (1888). The diagnosis of pericaecal abscess, and its radical treatment by removal of the appendix vermiformis. *J. Amer. med. Ass.,* 10, 733–9.

Morton, W. E. & Hahn, L. A. (1966). Epidemiology of congenital heart disease. *J. Amer. med. Ass.,* 195, 1107–10.

Nadler, H. L. & Gerbie, A. B. (1970). Role of amniocentesis in the intra-uterine detection of genetic disorders. *New Engl. J. Med.,* 282, 596–99.

Naidoo, S. (1972). *Specific dyslexia.* Pitman, London.

NCB (1972). *From birth to seven.* Longman, London.

Neligan, G. A. & Harris, M. (1965). See *Paediatrics in the Seventies,* ed. D. Court & A. Jackson. OUP, p. 6.

Neville, B. G. R., Harris, R. F., Stern, D. J. & Stern, J. (1971). Maternal histidinaemia. *Arch. Dis. Childh.,* 46, 119–21.

Newcastle ASB group (1975). Asymptomatic bacteriuria in schoolchildren in Newcastle upon Tyne. *Arch. Dis. Childh.,* 50, 90–102.

O'Brien, J. S., Okada, S., Chen, A. & Fillesup, D. L. (1970). Tay-Sachs disease detection of heterozygotes and homozygotes by serum hexosaminidase assay. *New Engl. J. Med.,* 283, 15–20.

Oppé, T. E. (1964). Medical problems of coloured immigrant children in Britain. *Proc. roy. Soc. Med.,* 57, 321–3.

Parkin, M. (1972–3). Disorders of growth in Medicine No. 2. *Endocrine Diseases,* ed. S. Campbell-Smith.

Parkin, M. (1975). Personal communication.

Parsons, J. G. (1972). Assessment of attitudes in young people of school-leaving age handicapped by hydrocephalus or spina bifida cystica. *Develop. Med. Child Neurol.*, 14, supp. 27, 101–8.

Peel, Sir J. H. (1970). Domiciliary midwifery and maternity bed needs. HMSO, London.

Penick, S. B. & Stunkard, A. J. (1972). The treatment of obesity. In Reichsman, F. (1972), p. 226.

Pollitt, E. & Money, J. (1964 & 1966). Studies in the psychology of dwarfism. *J. Pediat.*, 64, 415 & 66, 381.

Powell, G. F., Brasel, J. A. & Blizzard, R. M. (1967). Emotional deprivation and growth retardation simulating idiopathic hypopituitarism. *New Engl. J. Med.*, 276, 1271–83.

Pringle, M. L. K. (1965). *Deprivation and education.* Longman, London.

Pryse-Phillips, W. E. (1969). *Epilepsy.* Wright, Bristol.

Quirk, R. (1972). *Speech therapy services.* DES, London.

Record, R. G. & Edwards, J. H. (1958). Environmental influences related to the aetiology of congenital dislocation of the hip. *Brit. J. prev. Soc. Med.*, 12, 8–22.

Registrar-general (1839). *First annual report of the Registrar-general of births, deaths and marriages in England.* Clowes, London.

Registrar-general (1923). *The Registrar-general's statistical review of England and Wales, for the year 1921.* New annual series, HMSO, London.

Reichert, P. (1973). Automation in medicine. *Documenta geigy.*

Reichsman, F. (1972). Ed. Advances in psychosomatic medicine, vol. 7. *Hunger and satiety in health and disease.* Karger, Basel.

Reid, J. J. A. (1969). *People with epilepsy.* HMSO, London.

Report (1972). *On confidential enquiries into maternal deaths in England & Wales 1967–69.* No. 1 Reports on Health and Social Subjects. HMSO, London.

Richards, I. D. G. & McIntosh, H. T. (1972). Confidential inquiry into 226 consecutive infant deaths. *Arch. Dis. Childh.*, 47, 697–706.

Roberts, J. R. & Watson, B. W. (1973). The objective assessment of hearing in the young infant. *Minerva Otorinolaring.*, 23, 188–96.

Robinson, M. J. & Norman, A. P. (1975). Life tables for cystic fibrosis. *Arch. Dis. Childh.*, 50, 962–5.

Roskies, E. (1972). *Abnormality and normality the mothering of thalidomide children.* Cornell U. Press, Ithaca & London.

Royal College of Physicians (1976). *Fluoride, teeth and health.* Pitman, London.

Rutter, M. (1970). *A neuro-psychiatric study in childhood.* Clinics in Developmental Medicine, Heinemann, London, Nos. 35/36.

Rutter, M., Tizard, J. & Whitmore, K. (1970). *Education, health and behaviour.* Longman, London.

Savage, D. C. L., Wilson, M. I., McHardy, M., Dewar, D. A. E. & Fee, W. M. (1973). Covert bacteriuria of childhood. A clinical and epidemiological study. *Arch. Dis. Childh.*, 48, 8–00.

Schenectady study (1949). *Cerebral palsy survey in Schenectady County.* N.Y. State Depts. Hlth., Educ., Mental Hygiene & Social Welfare.

Shackleton, C. H., Mitchell, F. L. & Farquhar, J. W. (1972). Difficulties in the diagnosis of the adrenogenital syndrome in infancy. *Pediatrics,* 49, 198–205.

Sharrard, W. J. W. (1971). *Paediatric orthopaedics and fractures.* Blackwell, Oxford.

Sheldon, Sir W. (1967). *Child welfare centres.* HMSO, London.

Sheridan, M. (1972). The reported incidence of hearing loss in children of seven years. *Develop. Med. Child Neurol.*, 14, 296–303.

Sheridan, M. (1973). Children of seven years with marked speech defect. *Brit. J. Disor. Commun.*, 8, 9–16.

Shields, J. R. (1972). An approach to therapy with immigrants. *Bulletin of the College of Speech Therapists,* 241.
Shih, V. E., Bixby, E. M., Alpers, D. H., Bartsocas, C. S. & Thier, S. O. (1971). Studies of intestinal transport defect in Hartnup disease. *Gastroenterology,* 61, 445–53.
Smith, J. M. (1961). Prevalence and natural history of asthma in school children. *Brit. med. J.,* 1, 711–13.
Sorsby, A. (1972). *The incidence and causes of blindness in England and Wales 1963–68.* Reports on Public Health and Medical Subjects No. 128. HMSO, London.
Spear, H. B. (1969). The growth of heroin addiction in the United Kingdom. *Brit. J. Addiction,* 69, 215.
Springett, V. H., Adams, J. C. S., D'Costa, T. B. & Hemming, M. (1958). Tuberculosis in immigrants in Birmingham, 1956–57. *Brit. J. prev. Soc. Med.,* 12, 135–40.
Springett, V. H. (1972). Tuberculosis epidemiology in England and Wales. *Brit. med. J.,* 1, 422–3.
Sterky, K. (1963). Diabetic schoolchildren. *Acta paediat.* (Uppsala), supp. 144.
Stroud, C. E. (1971). Nutrition and the immigrant. *Brit. J. Hosp. Med.,* 5, 629–34.
Summerfield, A. (1968). *Psychologists in education services.* DES, HMSO, London.
Swan, C. H. J. & Cooke, W. T. (1971). Nutritional osteomalacia in immigrants in an urban community. *Lancet,* 2, 456–9.
Tanner, J. M., Goldstein, H. & Whitehouse, R. H. (1970). Standards for children's height at ages 2–9 years allowing for height of parents. *Arch. Dis. Childh.,* 45, 755–62
Taylor, N. R. W. (1972). Malignant disease in childhood. *Health Trends,* 4, 59–60.
Thalhammer, O. (1970). Histidinaemia detected by newborn screening using Guthrie's method. *Arch. Dis. Childh.,* 40, 820.
Theime, W. T., Wynne-Davies, R., Blair, H. A. F., Bell, E. T. & Loraine, J. A. (1968). Clinical examination and urinary oestrogen assays in newborn children with congenital dislocation of the hip. *J. Bone Jt. Surg.,* 50B, 546–9.
Tizard, J. (1958). *Mental deficiency: the changing outlook.* Methuen, London.
Treves, F. (1888). Relapsing typhlitis treated by operation. *Med.-chir. Trans.,* 71, 165–72.
Turk, J. (1964). Impact of cystic fibrosis on family functioning. *Pediatrics,* 34, 67–71.
Vaishnava, H. & Rizvi, S. N. A. (1971). Nutritional osteomalacia in immigrants in an urban community. *Lancet,* 2, 1147–8.
Valdes-Dapena, M. A. (1967). Sudden and unexpected death in infancy: a review of the world literature 1954-66. *Pediatrics,* 39, 123–38.
Vaughan, D. H. (1968). Families experiencing a sudden, unexpected infant death. *J. Roy. Coll. gen. Practit.,* 16, 359–67.
Vernon, M. (1972). *The education of the visually handicapped.* HMSO, London.
Watson, H. (1968), *Ed. Paediatric cardiology.* Lloyd-Luke, London, p. 71.
Widdowson, E. M. (1948). Mental contentment and physical growth. *Lancet,* 1, 1316–00.
Wilcken, B. & Turner, B. (1973). Homocystinuria: reduced folate during pyridoxine treatment. *Arch. Dis. Childh.,* 48, 58–62.
Witzleben, C. L., Monteleone, J. A. & Rejent, A. J. (1972). Electron microscopy in the diagnosis of cystinosis. *Arch. Path.,* 94, 362–5.
Woods, G. (1963). A lowered incidence of infantile cerebral palsy. *Develop. Med. Child Neurol.,* 5, 449–50.
Wootton of Abinger, Baroness (1970). *Advisory Committee on drug dependence: the amphetamines and lysergic acid diethylamide.* HMSO, London.

Wynn, M. (1964). *Fatherless families.* Joseph, London.

Wynn, M. & Wynn, A. (1972). *Some consequences of induced abortion to children born subsequently.* Foundation for education and research in child-bearing, London.

Wynne-Davies, R. (1964). Talipes equino-varus, talipes calcaneo-valgus and metatarsus varus. *J. Bone Jt. Surg.,* 46B, 445–63.

Wynne-Davies, R. (1966). Scoliosis: a family survey. *Ibid.,* 48B, 583.

Wynne-Davies, R. (1968). Familial (idiopathic) scoliosis. *Ibid.,* 50B, 24.

Zacune, J. & Hensman, C. (1971). *Drugs, alcohol and tobacco in Britain.* Heinemann, London.

Index